HEAL HEMORRHOIDS THROUGH AYURVEDA

DR. VIVEKANAND MOHAN KULLOLLI
DR. KRISHNA THORAT KULLOLLI

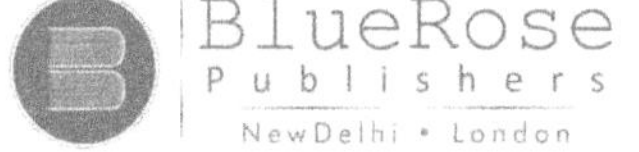
BlueRose Publishers
NewDelhi • London

First Published in January 2022

ISBN: 978-93-93388-95-7

BLUEROSE PUBLISHERS
www.bluerosepublishers.com
info@bluerosepublishers.com
+91 8882 898 898

Cover Design:
Aveek

Typographic Design:
Rohit

Distributed by: BlueRose, Amazon, Flipkart

Salutations

वक्रतुण्डो महाकायः कोटिसूर्यसमप्रभः ।
एकदंष्ट्रः कृष्णपिङ्गो विकटो धूम्रवर्णकः ॥ ९९॥

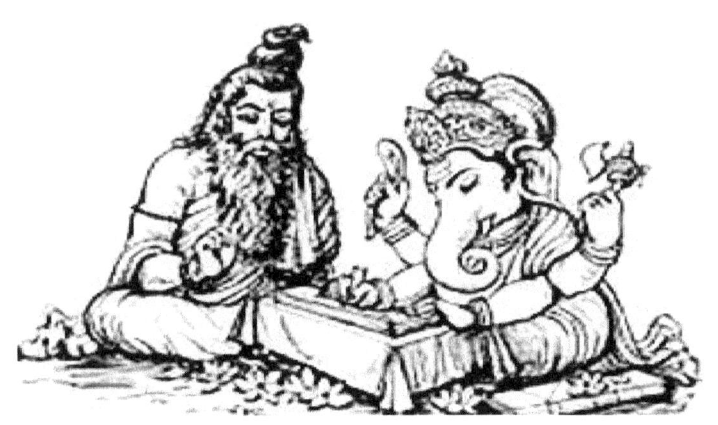

Dedication

Dedicated to The First Teachers, Friends, Care Takers and Inspirations of My Life, that is My Parents, Late **Shree. Mohan Kullolli** and Late **Shreemati. Mala Kullolli**, because of whom, I could survive and establish myself in this world and became able to give back to this Universe in the form of knowledge, that, I could acquire from all my teachers. I also dedicate this piece of work to you, one of my millions of readers, to add value to your life, who may be a student of Ayurveda, a Medical Practitioner or an inquisitive reader.

Acknowledgement

Expressing the gratitude is the simplest but more humble way of giving credit to the people, that are the reasons for the out come of this work. Without all of these, this book would not have been accomplished. The universe guides to do some work, and it only will arrange the modes and routes to accomplish the same, in the form of the people and events in our life.

I remember my parents and Sisters (Mrs. Veena and Mrs. Vidya) and acknowledge their support and the guidance throughout my learning in my life. I inherited the habit of reading variety of books from my father, Late Mr. Mohan Kullolli, who was A Librarian by Profession in a Degree college and was a voracious reader. My mother Mrs. Mala Kullolli, a secondary school teacher by profession, was my first teacher and given me the various lessons of the life and stood behind me as a Solid rock throughout my ups and downs of the life. I owe my achievements to them. My better half and the co-author of this book Dr. Krishna Thorat has been the constant inspiration and supporter for all my ventures, since the beginning of our relationship. Because of her sacrifices and love, I am free to think and create my books, to contribute for the readers world. Whenever I suffer with the procrastination, the sweet talks and smiles of my beautiful daughter, the little lioness, Ms. Vajraa and my nieces Ms. Neha and Ms. Shambhavi, gets me motivated and could accomplish this work.

When you are secured financially, then you could think of doing something extra. The constant support and motivation by my employers Dr. Devanshubhai Patel, The President, Parul University, Vadodara, India and other Trustees Dr. KomalBen Patel, Dr. GeethikaBen Patel and Dr. ParulBen Patel, has helped me to concentrate on creating this book.

My Guides and Mentors Dr. Prasanna Narasimha Rao, The Principal, S.D.M college of Ayurveda, Hassan, Karnataka, India and Dr. Hemanth Toshikhane, Dean, Faculty of Ayurved, Parul University, Vadodara, Gujarat, India, are always my inspirations, to aspire for more and add value for the society. I feel grateful to them for identifying the potentials and guiding me to the path of contribution to help the sufferers. I also thank them for their forewords.

All my teachers who taught me from the basic words to the much complex Ayurvedic science, will be the righteous owners of this work. I thank My Teachers Dr. Anand Sanakal, Former Principal, Ayurveda Maha Vidyalaya, Hubli, Karnataka, who taught me the basics and complex interpretations of the Ayurveda; Dr. P. Hemanth Kumar, Dean P.G. Studies and Head of the Department, National Institute of Ayurveda, Jaipur, India, who taught me the Surgery and provided the Forward For this book; Dr. Sekhar Nambudiri, Dr.S.K.Bannigol, Principal, Sanjeevini Ayurvedic Medical College Hubli and Former Head of the Department, Department of Shalya Tantra, Ayurveda Mahavidyalya Hubli; Dr.B.G.Kulkarni, Principal, Parul Institute of Ayurved and Research and all my Teachers of Ayurveda Maha Vidyalaya Hubli and S.D.M. College of Ayurveda, Hassan for their teachings and blessings.

I also express my gratitude to all my Colleagues and Post graduate scholars of Parul Institute of Ayurved, Parul University, Vadodara, Gujarat, India, for their constant support and help.

Last but not the least, I am grateful to all My patients, for their immense faith in my skills and knowledge, that has allowed me to understand and validate the Ayurveda principles in treating the cases of Haemorrhoids.

Foreword

I feel extremely happy to write foreword for the book entitled **"Heal Hemorrhoids Through Ayurveda"** by Dr Vivekanand Mohan Kullolli and Dr Krishna Thorat Kullolli. By considering the complexities faced by the scientific community and society in understanding the concepts of piles through *Samprapti Vighatana*, I could really sense that this piece of contribution will stand at its zenith. When I looked into the pages of the book, I could realize that the authors have carved out the book by touching the minds of common man in an understandable language with appropriate illustrations where ever applicable.

The finest berries of his multidimensional intellectual labour have been witnessed in his interpretation of the Ayurveda in terms of Haemorrhoids, stands in its own precise grade as the utmost legacy. I strongly believe such novel dimension thought provoking piece of work will undoubtedly bring a new outlook and insights to the young generation.

I hope this work will be highly beneficial to the society, students, teachers and research aspirants. I believe the readers will find every page of this book rewarding and satisfying. Also, I am sure that that this edition will definitely find a wider reading public.

I congratulate the authors for this literary work in bringing out this book for the benefit of the society. I bless the authors for their prosperity in the life ahead and rendering my warm wishes for their future endeavours.

Dr Hemant D Toshikhane
M.S.(Ayu), Ph.D., MBA, LLB.
Dean, Faculty of Ayurveda
Parul University Vadodara
Gujarat India. &
The Author of "Sushrutha's Physics."

Foreword

I congratulate Dr. Vivekanand Kullolli and Dr. Krishna Thorat for their genuine work of **"Heal Hemorrhoids Through Ayurveda"** on the Hemorrhoids. I appreciate the finest work that has been done to evaluate the causes and the pathogenesis of the Piles. "*Nidana Parivarjana meva Sankshepataha Chikitsa*", so, the basic treatment of any disease is to avoiding its causative factors, before advancing into the actual treatment. This book gives you an insight towards the causes of the Haemorrhoids, so that mere avoiding those causes you can prevent the Haemorrhoids in you and also you can cure it if it is identified in the earliest stage.

The comparison that, the authors have established, out of their vast clinical experience, between the classical Ayurvedic types of Piles and the contemporary science, will help the readers and the budding Ayurvedic surgeons, to plan their treatment in more effective way.

The part one of this book is a pure classical treat, for those, that intend of helping the patients of haemorrhoids, through Ayurveda. The classical remedies that are available for the haemorrhoids, have been narrated with more précised cause and effect relationship. At the same time, The Second Part helps the readers to understand the Haemorrhoids and its treatment modalities available in the contemporary science. This exhibits the pure professional intentions and the humanely concerns of the authors to help the sufferers to find the right treatment with less risk and cost effectiveness near to them.

I appreciate the Third Part of this book, for its effort of summarizing the whole concept of the Piles and Haemorrhoids with the *Arsha* disease, in most simple way to help the common people to understand their disease and help themselves at the earliest, to prevent the surgery.

I feel and suggest that this book is the first of its kind to evaluate the Haemorrhoids in more classical way without any bias. And this will help the learners of Ayurveda and Surgery, to understand and explore the Haemorrhoids in better way towards managing it medically. I feel it will be a must-read reference book for all those who want to explore more about the Haemorrhoids.

I bless and wish them all the best for their future endeavors and pray the God Dhanvantari to bless the authors with better health and longevity to undertake many more such classical works for the Ayurveda Lovers.

Professor (Dr) Prasanna Narasimha Rao

M.S. (Ayurveda), Ph.D.

Principal

S.D.M college of Ayurveda and Hospital

Hassan, Karnataka.

Foreword

It gives me immense pleasure to endorse that, this book of **"Heal Hemorrhoids Through Ayurveda"** takes forward the understanding of Haemorrhoids from the point of view of Ayurveda in more subtle way. The read from this book will help the readers to understand the etiologies, pathogenesis and the remedies of Haemorrhoids in a better way, so that the best treatment modality can be selected.

The beauty of this book is that, it highlights **the preventive aspects** and **the preventive measures** of the Piles and also emphasis on the **medical management of the same**, if diagnosed early and implemented promptly.

The need of the hour is to bridge the gap between the Ayurveda and the Modern medical science to serve the mankind, with holistic approach. Every science has its own strength and the limitation. If all the available medical sciences are looked into with the intention of strengthening each other in the good interest of the mankind, then wonders can be done. And this book is beautifully crafted to serve this purpose. The book gives the detail description about the *Arsha* and the Haemorrhoids, as it is in the respective science, without any bias, and leaves it to the privilege of the readers to have their interpretations and the conclusions about the disease.

The author has put all the essence of his clinical experience in the Part Three of this book. His approach towards the disease, makes him one of the best authorities, known for the medical management of the *Arsha*. The read of this section is a must for all the Shalya Tantra postgraduates and the Ayurvedic surgeons, even though this section is dedicated to the common non-medical people.

Every chapter of this book is a building block of this well-crafted book with the 'Prologue', "Some Basics of Ayurveda for the Beginners" and the 'Epilogue' being the important corner stones. I believe that both the Pro-Ayurvedic as well as non-Ayurvedic readers will equally cherish and will be benefitted by the golden nuggets of this book, because of its easy language and relevant explanation in English and Modern medical science. I feel that the primary reading of this book will help the readers to understand and implement the measures of my book, "Recent Trends in The Management of Arshas / Haemorrhoids," in better way in their clinical practice.

So, I congratulate and wish all the best for the future endeavors of these authors, expecting more such classical works from the author duos.

Professor (Dr.) P. Hemantha Kumar
M.S. (Ayu), Ph.D.
Dean (PG Studies)
Head of the Department
Department of Shalya Tantra
National Institute of Ayurveda
Jaipur, India.

Contents

Prologue

When, I thought of writing this book, I had the only intention of sharing my understanding about the most common disease, **The Haemorrhoids**. In last twenty plus years of my clinical practice, I could feel the pain and worries of all my patients about their illness. Most of them were apprehensive about this disease, because of involvement of their most fragile and private part. Their apprehension was the result of their misconception or wrong guidance from their nearest pal or unfortunately, some times by their non expert (non experty about the Ano-Rectal Diseases) family doctors. Even then, many a times, the apprehension is good enough to drive the patient to the concerned experts at the earliest. But, negligence of patient as well as their first attending doctors, many a times, lands the patient to the Surgery.

Surgery can be avoided, if the attending doctor gives an extra ounce over the complaints. It is my common observation that, at least nine out of ten general medical practitioners, will prescribe the medicines, without making an effort to examine the Anus and the Rectum, the site of the disease. It is also a common myth among many, especially, the common people that, any problem or pain at their Anus and buttocks, is due to Haemorrhoids. Unfortunately, the Anus can be the seat for many other pathological conditions. Fissure-in-Ano, Fistula-in-Ano, Perianal Abscesses, Anal Warts, Hypertrophied Anal Papillae and the life-threatening Cancerous growths or Tumors, can affect the Anal region.

Many a times, I felt that, if the patient would have come a little bit early, then I could have saved them from the painful surgery. The long-lasting list of wonderful Ayurvedic medicines, could have given them the better relief and prevention from these Piles. The fear and hesitancy of the patients, results into the late or wrong diagnosis, which complicates the course of the disease. As J.

Goligher JC quotes that, every individual, will suffer from Piles at least once in his life time[1] and fifty percent of the population have these Piles before they could reach their fifties. So, now you can feel the gravity and the incidence of the disease.

Even though, there are many books, already in the Universal Library on the Piles & Haemorrhoids, written by my respected Ayurvedic colleagues, I want to share my understanding about the Haemorrhoids, derived out of my clinical experiences. I hope, this book will help you to explore, the concept of Haemorrhoids with respect to its diagnosis and the treatment, that has been elaborated in Ayurveda, but unfortunately not much put into the practice.

The *Arsha,* that is how the Haemorrhoids/ Piles are referred in Ayurveda, share this name with other diseases, presenting with the ball like projections or abnormal growths. Arsha and its concepts can be attributed to the Piles, Haemorrhoids, Hypertrophied Anal Papillae, Anal Warts, Rectal Polyps and even to the Malignant Neoplasia of the Anal canal and the Rectum. But, considering the more common incidence of the Piles/Haemorrhoids, this book is focused on the Prevention and Cure of the Haemorrhoids.

My clinical experience, has always emphasized my inner voice, about the need of educating the sufferers as well as their negligent health care takers, regarding the importance of early detection and medicinal management of the Haemorrhoids. Also, by practicing Ayurveda way of life, the Piles can be prevented in majority of the population. Ayurveda, the science of life, has all the measures of preventions, management and cure of the disease. But unfortunately, it is less explored and used, even by its stakeholders. At the same time, it is my unfortunate finding that (with all my due respect to my contemporary fellow colleagues,), the preventive medicine for the Piles is either missing in western medicine or it is not given much ounce during the initial stage of the pathology. Ayurvedic medicines can be of great help to cure the Piles at the first and the initial stage of second degree, without any invasive procedures. So, the sole intention of this book is to give some glimpses of such medicines, dietary habits and diagnostic tips for prevention, early detection and cure with medical management, through Ayurveda.

The biggest challenge of crafting this book was, to make it readable and acceptable to general readers and non Ayurvedic medical professionals from the western world. For them, I have tried my level best to explain the Ayurvedic purview of hemorrhoids, with nearest Modern Medical Science words, wherever relevant, in the Part One of this book. My Ayurvedic colleagues, may feel it a repetitive reading for them. But, this way of presentation was inevitable as the intention of this book is to bridge the gap between the Ayurvedic Science and the Modern Medical Science, about the Haemorrhoids/ Piles. **"Some Basics of Ayurveda for the Beginners"** is an important chapter of this book about the basics of Ayurveda, with its nearest possible counterpart concepts of Modern Medical science, to understand the disease in a better way, so that every body gets value out of it. Hope, this chapter will help you to understand the First Part of this book, as if, you are a Pro Learner of the Ayurveda.

This book is divided into Three parts. The First Part is purely, the classical way of understanding the disease Haemorrhoids/Piles in terms of *Arsha*, counterpart of hemorrhoids / Piles in Ayurveda. This part may be felt difficult to read and understand by the non Ayurvedic readers, as I tried to explain the disease totally in Ayurveda way. But I tried to use most relevant and nearest meanings or words into the bracket next to the Sanskrit words. The Sanskrit words are highlighted by the Italic font and the first alphabet of the word in upper case, for easy identification. Hope, the patient reading will enable everyone to understand the concepts. It has been tried to explore and analyze, the minute and subtle concepts of the disease pathogenesis and its associated sequelae, in the form of the *Nidana Panchaka (The five Basic pillars of the manifestation of the disease pathology).*

1. The *Hetu* (Etiology), are the reasons or causes for the disease. It has got its own subclassification based on the factors involved. The most influencing factors on our body, mind, sense organs and soul, can be the reason for the disease, if they conjugate with our body in improper and abnormal proportion.

2. The *Samprapti* (Pathophysiology), deals with the stages of the manifestation of the diseases, right from its nidus of origin to its preclinical stage to clinical stage and its complications. The, in-depth evaluation of the *Samprqpti* will help the clinician, to assess the strength of the patient to tolerate the medicines, procedures (surgical/ para surgical/ panchakarma therapies) and the impact of the disease.

3. The *Poorvaroopa* (The Prodromal Signs & Symptoms) help to identify the disease, before its full manifestation stage and by that, the clinician can prevent the progress of the pathology to the clinical stage. Medicinal management of the Piles has got best result in this stage.

4. The *Roopa* (The Clinical stage), patient usually comes in this stage to his doctor. This is the stage of complete manifestation of the disease. Most of the signs and symptoms become evident as the pathology is localized to a particular part, organ or system of the body. Depending upon the clinical stage of the disease, the management is planned. The treatment varies from Medicine Management (when it is non prolapsing) to surgical or para-surgical intervention, when it becomes prolapsed.

5. The *Upashaya & Anupashaya* (The Pacifying & Aggravating Factors); The unique Ayurvedic way of testing the subtle factors of the disease pathology, enables to understand the involvement of the basic factors of the disease production i.e., the *Dosha* (basic Constituents of the body that maintain the normal physiology, when they are in their normalcy and produce the diseases, when they are vitiated).

The Second Part is regarding the description about the Piles (When, it is Non- bleeding)/ Haemorrhoids (when, it is bleeding) and its pathology and managements. This Part will help you to understand the disease with contemporary science perspective. As, the medicine management is limited from the modern Allopathic Science, the surgical procedures that are used, are highlighted more.

The Third Part is for all, who are from all the three categories, to whom this book is focused, that is, Ayurvedic learners & Practitioners, Allopathic Practitioners and The Common people, who do not have any medical knowledge and may be suffering with the Haemorrhoids or curious to know about the disease. In this, I have put all my clinical experiences to make this section worth reading. I have tried my level best to simplify the medical terminologies to make it easy for all to understand and implement the advises and use the medications to cure the Haemorrhoids. The book is concluded with my clinical understanding of the disease and final suggestions to all my readers to draw the final picture of the disease, in the epilogue.

If you are able to understand, some common Medical and Biological words, then read the Second Part first, then come back to the First Part, that should make you to understand the disease concept in Ayurveda more clearly. If, you do not want to know much about Ayurveda and want a ready to use prescription with respect to the medication and the compatible diet for the disease, then I believe that the Third Part should be an easy go through for you.

Some Basics of Ayurveda for the Beginners

As, this book is aimed to help all the people, right from an Ayurvedic Practitioners to the one who is unaware about the Ayurveda, this section is provided to help to understand some basics concepts of Ayurveda. Once you read this section, I believe that, you will be able to understand the whole disease process of the Haemorrhoids and the principles used to treat it, as per Ayurveda. Even, if you are here, out of some curiosity to know about the Ayurveda and its remedies for the Haemorrhoids, you will be able to read other Ayurvedic books with an ease. Even though it is difficult to summarize the whole concepts of the Ayurveda in one-chapter, best efforts are made here to give you the most solid basics of Ayurveda in the language of modern science, so that even non Ayurvedic persons can understand it. So, start your journey through the world's oldest life Science, the nature's own Medical Care.

What is Ayurveda?

Ayurveda is composed of two *Sanskrit* words, meaning of two words combined as '*Ayu*' *meaning* 'Life Span' and the '*Veda*' meaning 'Science'. So, it is a life science believed to be before the start of the Human life on the earth. *Veda*, the oldest scripts dated back to the time immemorable, describe that, as the lactation (production of milk) starts before the birth of the child, the Ayurveda was created by the Lord Bramha, (The God of Creation) for the welfare of the human species, well before its origin on the earth. But this medicine was materialized by God Dhanvantari (The God of Nectar). It was earlier used for the Gods, by the Ashwini Devata (the twin brothers, known as the physicians of the Devine Territory).

This wisdom of life science was received by Sage *Bharadwaj*, King *Deodasa Dhanvantari* (other than the God Dhanvantari) and sage *Kashyap* from the God Indra and developed the science into different branches. The medicine branch was developed by the Sage Bharadwaj, the surgical branch was developed by the King Deodasa Dhanvantari and the pediatrics branch was developed by the Sage Kashyapa. Further, their disciples developed the existing eight branches of the Ayurveda that are 1. *Kaya Chikitasa* (Internal Medicine), 2. *Bala Roga* (Pediatrics, Gynecology and Obstetrics), 3. *Jara Chikitsa / Rasayana* (Gerontology), 4. *Vrashan / Vajikarana* (Aphrodisiacs), 5. *Damshtra Chikitsa / Agada Tantra* (Toxicology and treatment of the poisons), 6. *Bhoota Vidya / Graha Bada* (Treatment of Super natural powers and microbes), 7. *Shalya Tantra* (Surgery and Para surgical treatment) and 8. *Shalakya Tantra / Urdhwanga Chikitsa* (Ear, Nose, Throat, Eyes and Dentistry).

The Ayurveda has got well developed Herbal, Animal, Herbo-Mineral and Mineral drug formularies developed over the time to treat the diseases without surgery. The *Sushruta*, is known as the father of the Surgery for his first ever contribution about the plastic surgery, laparotomy and other general surgical methods and the first person to explain about the Human Dead Body Dissection to explore the Human Anatomy, now explored by the modern anatomist, almost the same.

The *Charak*, known as the best physician has given the remedies of internal medicine in two categories like 1. Suppression of the *Dosha* (humors) called as *Shamana Chikitsa*, when *Dosha* are vitiated by their qualities or functions and 2. Drainage of *Dosha* (humors) called as *Shodhana Chikitsa*, if their toxic effects are because of increase of their quantity. The toxic *Dosha* are drained out of the body through the unique treatment methodology called the *Panchakarma* (The Five Types of Drainage Procedures).

The Ayurveda is based on the *Panchaboutika Siddhant* (Five Basic Elemental Theory); *Tridosha Siddhant* (Three Humoral Theory); *Karya- Karana Siddhant* (The Cause & Effect Theory); *Samanya- Vishesha Siddhant* (Similarity & Dissimilarity Theory) and *Loka- Purusha Sadharmya Siddhant* (Similarity of the external world and internal environment of the body Theory).

1. **The *Panchaboutika Siddhant* (Five Basic Elemental Theory) and *Loka-Purusha Sadharmya Siddhant* (Similarity of the external world and internal environment of the body Theory):**

   It is undisputed that, this universe is having basic five elements of Earth, Water, Fire, Air and Aether as its basis. Every object in the universe is the resultant of the varying composition of all these five elements.

   The Earth is known as *Prithvi* in Sanskrit, helps to give solid structure and shape to the objects, let it be animate or inanimate. It's the main composition of Bones, Muscles, Tendons, Ligaments, Capsules, Soft Tissues and organs like Liver, Kidney, Intestines, Vessels etc.

   The water element known as the *Aap /Jala/ Ambu* helps to form all the liquid tissues and waste products in the body, like Lymph, Blood, Cerebro- Spinal Fluid, Synovial Fluids, Digestive Juices, Sweat and Urine etc.

   The Fire element is *Agni* of three main types i.e., *Jatharagni* (Gastric, Biliary, Pancreatic and Intestinal Juices), *Dhatavagni* (Digestive Enzymes at Tissue level) and the *Bootagni* (Metabolic Enzymes at the Cellular Level).

   The Air element is Named as *Vata / Vayu / Sameera / Pavana* and is meant for the transmission of neuro-electrical impulses to create the movement and sensory perception of the body and its physiology. Whereas, the Aether is known as the *Akasha*, responsible to crate the space and cavity inside the body for the easy accommodation of the organs and movement of the solid, liquid and gaseous materials.

   This similarity of the bodily tissues with the basic characters of the five elements, that can be visualized and pursued in the exterior world, itself is known as the *Loka- Purusha Sadharmya*

Siddhant, used to compensate the loss of the same in the body from external supplementation. All the objects, both animate and inanimate are having all the five elements in their compositions, but based on the predominance of one of the elements, they are named as either *Parthivya* (Earth Predominant), *Aapya* (Water Predominant), *Aagneya* (Fire Predominant), *Vayuvya* (Air Predominant) and *Aakasheeya* (Aether Predominant). This variation in the composition of the percentage of the elements is termed as *Tara-Tama Bhava* in Ayurveda. *Tara* being the small fraction compared to the *Tama Bhava,* that happens to be the biggest fraction or portion of the particular combination. This *Tara-Tama Bhava* is particularly used to denote the percentage of vitiation of the *Dosha* (Humors), in the disease process, when all the three *Dosha* are involved. For example, it may be denoted as Vata Dosha-Pitta Tara-Kapha Tama, indicating the ascending order of vitiation of the Dosha in percentage to contribute for the disease pathology. Here, *Vata Dosha* is involved in least percentage while, *Pitta Dosha* is in more percentage compared to the *Vata Dosha* and in less percentage compared to the *Kapha Dosha.*

2. ***Tridosha Siddhant* (Three Humoral Theory)**: The *Tri* denotes the number Three and the *Dosha* denote the basic functional units of the body, the Humors. The word Humor may not be the exact word to describe the overall features of the *Dosha*, but that is the word used by my predecessors to denote the *Dosha.* So, the same word from the English language, we will use to refer to the *Dosha* here in further. As the number denotes, they are three, 1. *Vata / Vayu* (Air+Aether elements), 2. *Pitta* (Fire+Water elements) and 3. *Kapha /Shleshma* (Earth +Water elements). Their actions both physiological and pathological, depend upon their properties, that are derived from the compositions of their basic elements, as mentioned in the bracket, in front of each of them.

The *Vata*, has got the Six Properties viz, 1. *Ruksha* (Dry), 2. *Sheeta* (Cold), 3. *Laghu* (Lightness), 4. *Khara* (Rough), 5.

Sukshma (Fine/ Invisible/ Subtle) and the most important one is 6. *Chala* (Movement). If any abnormal change, in any of these properties either quantitatively, qualitatively or functionally will lead to the onset of the disease pathogenesis. Because of its properties, the *Vata* simulates much with the Boney Structures and Its Cavities, so the *Asthi* (The Bone) happens to be the shelter for the *Vata Dosha*, among the Seven *Dhatu* (meaning giving shelter to or withholding; and Tissues can be referred to as *Dhatu*). This phenomenon of Sheltering the *Dosha* in *Dhatu* is called as *Dosha-Dooshya (Dhatu) Ashrayashrayeebhava*. So, the treatment aimed at *Vata* will have positive effect on the Bone Also. So, the properties similar to the properties of *Vata* and *Rasa* (Taste) of foods like *Katu* (Pungent), *Tikta* (Bitter) and *Kashaya* (Astringent) will aggravate it and the opposite properties like *Snigdha* (Unctuousness), *Ushna* (Hot), *Guru* (Heavyness), *Shlakshna* (Smooth), *Sthoola* (wide/ broad/ obese), *Sthira* (firm) and the Taste like *Madhura* (Sweet), *Amla* (Sour), *Lavana* (Salt) and objects with Hot potency (*Ushna Veerya*) and heat will suppress or pacify the *Vata*.

The *Vata*, is having its 5 sub types assigned for different physiological functions in the body. 1. *Prana Vata*, located in the upper half of the body and takes care of the inspiration, deglutination, intellectual thinking and all brain and cranial nerves functions. 2.*Udana Vata*, also located in the upper half of the body and takes care of expiration, spitting, burping, motivation, initiation, expressions etc. all outward movements from the body and functions of spinal nerves of upper half of the body 3. *Samana Vata* is in the upper and mid gut, facilitates, the peristaltic movements of the intestines and the free flow of the Gastric, Biliary, Pancreatic and Intestinal Juices and secretions to help in the digestion, through splanchnic and mesenteric nerve plexuses. 4. *Vyana Vata* seated at the Heart and its Vascular networks and takes care of the Cardiovascular System. 5. *Apana Vata*, most dominant among the five and influences the other four *Vata*, as per its status. This is like the head of all the other *Vata* to control all the bodily functions of the whole Nervous System. It's mainly centered at the Lower half of the body, large colon, genitalia, urinary system and legs. Lumbar,

Sacral and Coccygeal plexuses of the spinal nerves and Vagus nerve come under the functional domain of the *Apana Vata*. The locomotory functions of legs, excretion of urine, feces and flatus, discharge of menstrual fluids, ejaculation of the semen and expulsion of fetus are attributed to the functions of *Apana Vata* along with maintaining of other four *Vata*.

The *Vata* imparts black, brick red, bluish -black colours to the parts and contents of the body, in its pathological status, along with emaciation of the tissues and body, tremors and most importantly the Pain. The pain is the hallmark of the vitiation of the *Vata Dosha*, which is most often characterized by pricking type of Pain.

The *Pitta*, takes care of all the digestion, conversion and metabolisms, at both in the gut and at the cellular level. It's five types take care of different functions at different levels. 1. *Pachaka Pitta*, is in the gut, and constituted by all the secretions of Biliary, Pancreatic and Intestinal parts. It takes care of the main digestion at the macro level. It is the main *Pitta* and has got it's influence on the rest of four other *Pitta*. 2. *Ranjaka Pitta*, is at the stomach and also at the liver and spleen, taking care of the conversion of the exogenous hematinic materials into the endogenous forms of the Blood components. 3.*Sadaka Pitta*, resides in the Heart and helps for the courage and decision-making ability. 4.*Alochaka Pitta*, is in the eyes and helps for the vision acuity, the vitreous and aqueous humor composition and physiology is dependent on the *Alochaka Pitta*.5. *Bhrajaka Pitta*, takes care of the skin metabolism and its maintenance.

The *Pitta* is sheltered in the *Rakta* (Blood). So, the physiology and pathology of both, remain same and are influenced by the same factors. Even though, physiologically, the *Pitta* has got light yellow colour, during its pathological state it imparts yellow colour to the skin, sclera in the eyes, nails, mucosa, bodily discharges and even to the urine and feces. It is the reason for the inflammation, burning sensation, bleeding pathologies and suppurations in the diseases.

The *Pitta* has got the properties of 1. *Sasneha* (Unctuousness), 2. *Teekshna* (Sharp and Penetrating), 3. *Ushnam* (Hot/Heat), 4.

Laghu (Lightness), 5. *Visram* (Foul odor), 6. *Saram* (Flowing), 7. *Dravam* (Liquidity). And any act or consumption of the drugs or foods of these properties and *Rasa* (Taste) like *Amla* (Sour), *Lavana* (Salt) and *Katu* (Pungent) will aggravate the *Pitta Dosha*. Opposite of these properties like *Ruksha* (Dryness), *Manda* (Slowness), *Sheeta* (Cold), *Guru* (Heavyness) with *Sheeta Veerya* (Cold Potency) and the *Rasa* (Taste) of *Madhura* (Sweet), *Tikta* (Bitter) and *Kashaya* (Astringent) will Pacify the *Pitta Dosha*.

The Kapha Dosha, is concerned with the repair, building and lubrication of the body. It is also of five varieties, 1. *Avalambhaka Kapha*, is in the thorax region and takes care of all the smooth functioning of the thoracic organs like lungs, heart and mediastinal structures. The normal mucosal secretions, pleural fluid and pericardial fluids are superficially considered as the variety of the *Avalambhaka Kapha*. It is the main *Kapha* to influence and maintain the status of the other four *Kapha*. 2. *Kledaka Kapha*.is considered as the mucous content of the gastric secretions. It helps in moistening the food and protects the gastrum from acid injury by creating the mucosal barrier over the mucosal layer of the stomach. 3. *Bodhaka Kapha*, is having its location at the tongue and oral cavity and helps to assess the taste and takes care of the moistening of the food bolus and it's easy churning. 4. *Shleshaka Kapha*, is in the joint spaces and meant for the easy lubrication and movement. Whereas, 5. *Tarpaka Kapha* is considered to be at the skull region and can be compared to the cerebro-spinal fluid.

The *Kapha Dosha* has got its properties like *Snigdha* (Unctuous), *Guru* (Heavy), *Sthira* (Stable), *Sheeta* (Cold), *Picchilam* (viscous) etc. and it is responsible for the Itching, Heaviness, Swelling and Pale color of the affected part, when it turns pathological. Kapha is sheltered in the rest of the five *Dhatus* i.e., *Rasa* (Chyle/ Lymph/ Serum/ Plasma), *Mamsa* (Muscle and its tendons), *Medh* (Adipose tissue), *Majja* (bone marrow and brain tissue) and *Shukra* (Semen and gonadotropins). And the treatment aimed at the *Kapha Dosha* will cure the diseases of these *Dhatu*, and vice versa.

3. ***Sapta Dhatu and ThreeMala*:** The body is made up of the seven *Dhatu* or tissues as 1. *Rasa* (Chyle/ Lymph/ Serum/ Plasma) is composed of *Aap Mahabhoota* (Water Element), it circulates nutrients, hormones and proteins throughout the body. 2. *Rakta* (Blood) with fire element in predominance followed by water Element 3. *Mamsa* (Muscle and its Tendons) composed of earth predominantly along with water elements, 4. Medh (Adipose tissue) is predominant of water element followed by earth element, 5. *Asthi* (The Bone) more predominant with the earth element followed by air element, that makes the bone sturdy and the cavity also. 6. *Majja* (bone marrow and brain tissue), that supports the bones and joints, is predominant of water element and is same with the 7. *Shukra Dhatu* (Semen).

4. The three major metabolic wastes are 1. *Pureesh /Shakrut / Vid /Vit* (Stools/ feces), is a solid waste predominant of earth element. 2. *Mootra* (Urine) is a liquid waste predominant of water elements. 3. *Sweda* (Sweat) predominant of water element followed by fire element. Even though, these are waste products, but before they are excreted out, they serve some necessary physiological functions like, a) providing strength to the spine, so that the person can stand erect, by the well-formed feces in the large colon; b) urine provides necessary hydration and maintains the homeostasis of the renal system throughout its course of passage. Whereas, the sweat maintains the normal hydration and texture of the skin to avoid Hyperthermia and the skin diseases.

Treatment Principles:

The Treatment for any disease can be achieved by the three measures, 1. Decreasing the abnormally increased *Dosha* and *Dushya* (*Dhatu* is termed as *Dushya* in the pathological state). 2. Increasing the decreased *Dosha* and *Dushya* and 3. Maintaining the status Co of the normal *Dosha* and *Dushya*.

The treatment principles are dependent on the Etiologies, Pathogenesis and the Tissues (Site of the disease) involved in the disease process. Once, these are identified with respect to which properties (*Guna*) of the *Dosha* and *Dushya* are vitiated, the *Samanya* (Similarity/ Similar properties)- *Vishesha* (Dissimilarity/ Dissimilar properties) Theory is applied to achieve any of the required objective of the above-mentioned treatment principles. The pathological increase of the *Dosha* can be reduced or pacified by applying the *Vishesha Siddhant*, that is using the food, medicine and the activities that possess the opposite properties of the increased *Dosha*. In case of pathologically decreased *Dosha*, the compensation is done from exterior source, in the form of food, medicines and activities that possess the similar properties as of the decreased *Dosha.* Usually, the increase in the *Dosha,* either Quantitative Increase (*Dravyata Vikruti)*, Qualitative Increase (*Gunataha Vikruti*) or Functional Increase (*Karmataha Vikruti*), are more potent to cause the disease compared to the decreased status of the *Dosha*. And, as the three *Dosha* possess majority of opposite properties among each other, usually permutation and combination of any of the two *Dosha* or all the three *Dosha* will be most of the time, with their similar or non-opposing properties. Whereas, prominent and distinct properties of each *Dosha* are mainly seen in the diseases produced because of the single *Dosha* (*Ekadoshaja*). If the combination of two (*Dwandva Dosha*) or Three *Dosha* (*Tridoshaja/ Sannipataja*) occurs with the involvement of all the properties of each *Dosha* involved, then the prognosis of the disease will be poor and many a times such diseases become difficult to cure or incurable.

'Without the Cause, there is no Effect' (Cause and Effect Relationship/ *Karya- Karana Sambhandha*). So, the diseases also will not occur without the etiologies. Moreover, the first line of the treatment is **"Avoidance of the Etiological Factors."** No treatment will be complete and effective without the avoidance of the causative factors. Detailed analysis of the causes of the disease, with respect to their properties (*Guna)*, that are aggravating the similar properties (*Samanya Guna*) of the *Dosha*, will help to come out with the most apparent and effective treatment plans, that will be comprised of the drugs and measures with the opposite properties (*Vishesha Guna*) of the aggravated *Dosha* and their respective Causes.

In three ways, we get afflicted by the diseases. 1. *Asatmendriyartha Samyoga*, 2. *Prajnyaparadha* and 3. *Parinama*.

1. *Asatmendriyartha Samyoga* is indulging into compatible as well as incompatible food, activities and the climatic changes. Excessive indulgence even in the compatible ones as well as minimal or untimely indulgence in incompatible stuffs, will cause the *Dosha* variation in the body to produce the disease.

2. *Prajnyaparadha* is knowingly indulging in the incompatible food, activities and exposing to the incompatible climate.

3. *Parinama* is the end result of the above two etiologies, that is the production of the effect of the indulgence in the incompatible stuffs.

So produced diseases, can be treated by Two main principles 1. *Vipareetakari Chikitsa* and 2. *Vipareetarthakari Chikitsa.*

1. *Vipareetakari Chikitsa* is treating the disease conditions by applying the measures and the medicines with the opposite properties of the causative factors and the diseases. Some of the conditions may require the treatment with the properties and the measures opposite to the properties of their causative factors. This is called as *Hetu Vipareetakari Chikitsa.* In the same way, when the treatment is planned with the opposite properties to the disease specific, then it is called as *Vyadhi Vipareetakari Chikitsa.* If, the treatment measures are opposite to both the causative factors and the disease, then it is called as the *Hetu-Vyadhi or Ubhaya Vipareetakari Chikitsa.*

2. *Vipareetarthakari Chikitsa* is treating either the causative factors or the disease specific or both with the measures and medicines of similar properties.

Vipareetakari Chikitsa is based on the Vishesha Siddhant whereas, Vipareetarthakari Chikitsa is applied with the Samanya Siddhant.

Hetu Vipareetakari Chikitsa is mainly achieved with either medicines or the Adravyabhoota chikitsa (without materials) like Daivavyapashraya (offerings to the God and Universe) and Satvavajaya (psychological counseling).

Vyadhi Vipareetakari Chikitsa can be achieved by either both by the medicines as well as the surgical procedures. Most of the surgical diseases require the Vyadhi Vipareetakari Chikitsa in the form of the surgical procedures.

Hetu-Vyadhi or Ubhaya Vipareetakari Chikitsa can be achieved by the Para-Surgical procedures like *Ksharakarma* (chemical cauterization by the herbal alkalis), *Agnikarma* (thermal cauterization) and Raktamokshana (blood letting therapies and Leech application).

The four-fold treatments mentioned for the Piles in Ayurveda depict all the three *Vipareetakari Chikitsa,* that is Bheshaja (medical management) for *Hetu Vipareetakari Chikitsa*; *Shastra Karma* (surgical management) for the *Vyadhi Vipareetakari Chikitsa* and *Kshara* and *Agnikarma* (para-surgical procedures) for the *Hetu Vyadhi Ubhaya Vipareetakari Chikitsa.*

Part One:
Review and Analyzations of Arsha (Haemorrhoids)

1 Vedic Over View of Arsha

Arsha (Piles), the disease characterized by the presentation of *Mamsankura (Flesh growth)* at the *Guda Bhaga* [2] (Anal Region), is the area of concern since the time immemorial. Because of its severity it is considered as one among the *Ashta Mahagada* (Eight Dreadful Diseases). Since it is difficult to treat completely because of its *Swabhava* (Nature) may cause problem to the patient as an enemy. Hence the name *Arsha* (Piles).

The word *Arsha* is derived from the '*Ru*' *Dhatu* with '*Asun Shru't pratyaya* which occurs at *Paayu (Anal Canal)*. Further, the word meaning points towards its nature of troubling the patient, as an enemy. It is popular with different names like *Durnamak* (having bad name as enemy), *Durnama* (bad name), *Gudakeela* (A pin or peg like tumour at anus), *Gudankura* (sprouts at anus), *Gudodbhava* (origins at anus) and *Anamakam* (infamous name).

Arsha has got its roots deep into the *Gambhira Dhatu (Deep and Vital Tissues)*. It originates from both the *Rakta Dhatu*[3] (Blood) as well as *Mamsa Dhatu*[4] (Muscle Tissue), when they are vitiated and get associated with all the *Tridosha* (The Three Humors of Body), with all their varieties. This indicates the *Bala* of the *Vyadhi* which has got 4-fold treatment as per the need i.e., *Bheshaja* (Medicament), *Shastra* (Surgery), *Kshara* (Alkali/ chemical cauterization) and *Agni* (Thermal Cautery/Red- hot Material application)

The 6 types of *Arsha* have got both *Bheshaja* and *Shastra karma* depending upon their extent of growth. *Arsha* finds its place both in the category of the *Chedhya* (Excisional) and *Lekhya Karma* (Scrapping / Curettage) among the *Ashtavida Shastra Karma* (Eight Types of Surgical Principles and Procedures). The

Ardra Arsha (Piles with discharge or / and Haemorrhoids) like *Pittaja* and *Raktaja Arsha* can be treated with *Kshara Karma* (Alkali both as External Application and internal Consumption), either by *Pratisarana* (Smearing, Alkali Paste) and or by *Kshara Sutra* (Medicated Thread- applied with Alkali and Latex), once they are not curable by the Bheshaja. Whereas, the *Shushka Arsha* (Dry, non-bleeding Piles) like *Vataja* and *Khapaja* are treated by the *Agni Karma* and *Kshara Karma*. *Agnikarma*, one of the *Anu Shastra* (Para Surgical Measure) is kept as the last option of the treatment modalities, among the 4, because of its ultimate effect, which does not allow the disease to reoccur. The *Sannipataja* (More Advanced Piles) and the *Sahaja* (Congenital) are considered to be *Asadhya* (Incurable).

The *Arsha* which can take shelter in both *Bahya Roga Marga* (Includes Limbs and External orifices like Eyes, Nose, Ears, Oral Cavity, Genito Urinary apertures and Anal orifice) and *Abhyantara Roga Marga* (occurring in Gastro Intestinal tract, Abdominal cavity & Thorax situated structures), has got different form of *Bheshaja Chikitsa*, especially the *Takra Prayoga* (Usage of Butter Milk) is highlighted with different combinations. Certain *Pathya* (Compatible regimen and diet with respect to, the control of the Disease) and *Apathya* (Incompatible regimen and diet with respect to, the control of the Disease) are specified to avoid the recurrence.

So, the *Arsha* which occurs at the *Guda Bhaga* is given more importance because of its severity, even though, it can occur in other places like *Nasa (Nasal cavity)*, *Gala (Throat)*, *Talu (Palate)*, *Mukha (Oral cavity)*, *Karna (Ears)*, *Nabhi (Umbilicus)*, *Akshivartma (Palabra / Eye lids)*, *Twak (Skin) and Apathypatha (Genito urinary Tract)*. *Mamsankura* occurring at *Guda* (Anal Canal) are termed as *Keela* and *Arsha*, whereas occurring in other places as the *Adimamsa*[5] (Skin Warts / Polyps / Stye / Rounded abnormal Growths). The *Arsha* is the condition, which causes much problem compared to the *Adimamsa*.

Incidence:

Arsha Roga (Piles Disease) being *Durnama*, doesn't spare any age group it seems. Because, it can occur along with the birth[6] also. It may trouble the human beings during the age to enter into *Grahasthashrama* (Active Familial & Sexual Life). Hence it is advised, as not to get marry, unless the person suffering from the *Arsha*, is cured off that disease[7]. More over the person of any age group, if doesn't follow the *Rutu Charya* (Seasonal Regimen advised in Ayurveda) and *Dinacharya* (Daily Regimen), and indulges in the *Nidana Sevana* (engages himself in the consumption of aetiological factors), may acquire the *Arsha*, as the *Janmottar Kalaja Vyadhi* (Acquired after the birth).

Sex incidence shows that, the males are much affected than the females. Because the *Nidana* that are responsible for the formation of *Arsha*, match with the life style of the males. Moreover, the girls are cautioned, as not to marry the man who is suffering with the *Arsha*[8]. But the females do suffer with the Arsha because of the either *Ama Garbha Patha* (miscarriages or abortions) or *Peedana (Pressure over the rectum and anal canal)* of the *Guda Bhaga* by the *Garbha* (Foetus) or because of *Vishama Prasuti* (Difficult Labour).

Avoiding the causative factors itself, can prevent the person from the disease. So, the knowledge of *Hetu (Aetiology)* is quite essential to advise the favourable regimen as the first line of treatment.

2

Hetu (Analyzation of Etiologies) of Arsha

The Sannikrishta Nidana (Direct Aetiologies) of Arsha i.e., Vata, Pitta and Kapha are vitiated due to the indulgence of the persons in the Viprakrishta Karana (Indirect or Supportive Causes) like the Ahara (Diet), Vihara (Regimen), Vrutti (Professional Causes) and changes in the day and season will definitely cause the manifestation of the disease of the Guda (Ana-rectal) i.e., Arsha (Piles).

The *Nidana of Arsha* (Aetiologies) can be classified in different categories to understand their immediate / late effect in the vitiation of the *Dosha* and to find out the *Nidana* for the *Khavaigunya* (Structural Changes in the channels of the body) and the role of the *Nidana (Causes)* in the manifestation of the *Samprapti* (Pathology). Since, the *Nidana is* classified under *Asatmendriyartha* (Improper or Incompatible Conjugation of influencing factors like Food, Habit, Daily Routines and Season/Climatic changes) etc, it is easy to give advice to the patient to avoid those causative factors. They are considered as following,

Table No.1: *Nidana for Vataja Arsha* [9]

Hethu bheda	Ahara	Vihara	Anya
Asatmendriyarth samyoga	Rasanendriya – • *Atiyoga – kashaya, katu, tikta rasa and shookadhanya* • *Mithya yoga – pramitashana* • *Heena yoga– alpashana*	*Sparshanendriya –* • *Ati yoga – sheeta desha and kala, atapa and vata sevana* • *Sheetambu prakshalana*	*Ubhayendriya –* • *Ati yoga – shoka*
Prajnyaparadha (Knowingly indulging in ill habits)	• *Atiyoga – kashaya katu tikta, rasa and shookadhanya; teekshna madhya pana* • *Mithya yoga – pramitashana; viruddha bhojana* • *Heena yoga – alpashana*	• *Ati yoga – sheeta desha and kala, atapa and vata sevana; maithuna, vyayama, langhana* • *Mithya yoga – utkatakasana; vishama kathinasana, vega vidarana, vega avarodha*	• *Ati yoga – shoka;* • *Mithya yoga – improper administration of basti netra*
Parinama (Effect of the Cause)	----------	---------	• *Ati yoga– of atapa in greeshma rutu* • *Mithya yoga – ati sheeta in varsha rutu*

Table No.2: *Nidana for Pittaja Arsha* [10]

Hethu bheda	Ahara	Vihara	Anya
Asatmendriyartha SamYoga	*Rasanendriya –* • *AtiYoga – lavana, kshara and katu rasa; vidahi anna, teekshna and ushna annapana, rasona, shukta sevana*	*SpArshanendriya –* • *Ati Yoga – ushna desha and kala, atapa and prabha sevana*	*Ubhayendriya –* • *Ati Yoga – krodha*
Prajnyaparadha	• *AtiYoga – lavana, kshara and katu rasa; teekshna madhya pana; vidahi ushna annapana; tila; dadisevana*	• *Ati Yoga – ushna desha and kala, atapa and prabha sevana and vyayama* • *Mithya Yoga – utkatakasana; Vishama Kathinasana, vega vidarana, vega avarodha*	• *Ati Yoga – krodha and asuyana*
Parinama	----	----	• *Ati Yoga – of ushnata in shishira rutu*

Table No.3: *Nidana for Khapaja Arsha* [11]

Hethu bheda	Ahara	Vihara	Anya
Asatmendriyartha SamYoga	*Rasanendriya* – • *AtiYoga – madhura, amla and lavana rasa; vishtambi anna, sheeta, snigdha and guru annapana,*	*SpArshanendriya* – • *Ati Yoga – sheeta desha and kala, pragVata sevana* • *Mithya Yoga – diva swapna* • *Heena Yoga - avyayama*	*Ubhayendriya* –
Prajnyaparadha	*AtiYoga – madhura, amla and lavana rasa; vishtambi anna, sheeta, snigdha and guru annapana;* *e.g., taruta, bisa, shaluka, krounydana, kasheruka, shrungataka etc., shaka;* *avi, varaha, gomamsa, mahisha mamsa, mathsya etc mamsa; ksheera, guru jalapana*	• *Ati Yoga – shayya sukha, sheeta desha and kala, pragVata* • *Mithya Yoga – diva swapna* • *Heena Yoga – avyayama*	• *Ati Yoga – achintana*
Parinama	----	----	• *Ati Yoga – of sheetata in hemanta rutu*

Along with these above-mentioned *Nidana*, the *Vyadhi Hethu* are common for all the types of *Arsha* which precipitate the condition. They are as follow:

Utkatakasana (Deep Squatting position), *Vishama Kathinasana* (Improper sitting on Hard and Rough Surfaces especially touching the Anus), *Avagharshana* (Rubbing) of *Guda Bhaga* (Anus) with *Sheetambu* (Extreme Cold Water), *Loshtra* (A type of Stone), Trina (Grass), *Pashana* (Stone); *Avyayama* (Not indulging any physical exercise), *Shayya Sukha* (Sedentary Life Style), improper administration of *Bastinetra* (Nozzle of Enema Pot).

In the same way the *Nidana (Aetiologies)* can be classified as *Sannikrishtadi* type as well as the *Dosha (Humor)*, *Vyadhi (Disease specific aetiology)* and *Ubhaya Hethu* (Both, Humor and Disease Specific aetiologies) type which will be more informative for the physician / surgeon to plan for his treatment.

Nidanartakara roga **(Secondary to Some Other Disease or Illness):** The disease *Atisara* (Diarrhoea), *Grahani* (irritable bowel syndrome; Ulcerative Colitis; Crohn's Disease) and *Arsha* are almost interrelated due to the common fact of *Agni Mandya* (Depressed Metabolism Rate) and one disease may cause the other. [12]

Other than these, the person who are emaciated due to the affection of the *Jwara* (Chronic Fever), *Gulma* (Tumours of Abdomen, both pseudo and organic), *Atisara*, *Ama* (Toxins in the Body; Improperly formed or Toxic Metabolites), *Grahani*, *Shoka* (Depression; Grief) and *Pandu* (Anaemia) may also suffer with the *Arsha*.[13]

Beeja dosha **(Inheritance or Genetic Cause):** Other than the *Bahya Karana*, the *Dosha* (Defect) in the *Beeja* (Gametes), can be as one of the major causes of Arsha especially *Sahaja Arsha* (Congenital Piles). The *Beeja Dosha* may be inherited through the *Matruja Beeja Bhagavayava* (Maternal chromosomes) or from the *Pitruja Beeja Bhagavayava* (Paternal Chromosomes), which is responsible for the defect in the formation of the *Gudavali* (Anal

Mucosal Folds). The *Beeja Dosha* (Defect in the Gametes), may be due to the *Apachara* (Improper) in the regimen of the father and mother or may be because of the *Purvakruta karma* (Attributed to the deeds of the previous life when the cause is untraceable / idiopathic). [14]

Fig. 1: NIDANA OF ARSHA

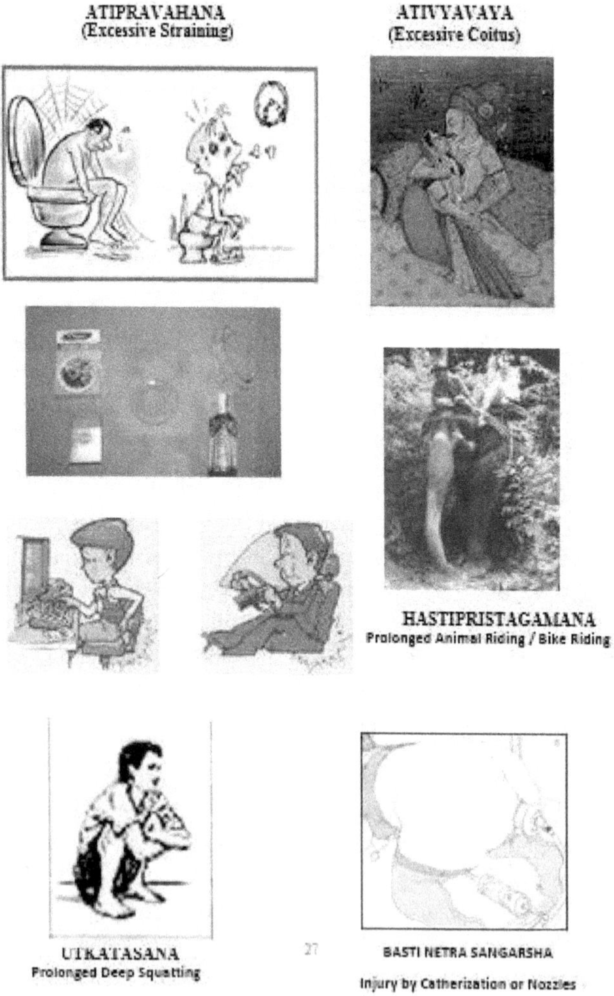

ATIPRAVAHANA
(Excessive Straining)

ATIVYAVAYA
(Excessive Coitus)

HASTIPRISTAGAMANA
Prolonged Animal Riding / Bike Riding

UTKATASANA
Prolonged Deep Squatting

27

BASTI NETRA SANGARSHA
Injury by Catherization or Nozzles

3
Samprapti (Analyzation of Pathophysiology) of Arsha

Samanya Samprapti (General Pathophysiology) [15]

The person having *Mandagni (Depressed Digestive Enzymes)*, either because of the *Vyadhi* like *Atisara*, *Grahani* etc., or due to the other causative factors, once indulges into the *Nidana sevana* (aetiologies), experiences the vitiation of the *Tridosha*, mainly *Vata*. The *Vata*, which starts moving in *Vimargagamana* (Opposite to its normal movements & directions), vitiates the other two *Dosha (The Kapha & The Pitta)*. So, these *Dosha* along with or without the association of the *Shonita* (Blood), start moving (*Prasara*) towards the *Guda Bhaga* (Ano-rectal region) through the 2 *Pureesha Vahi Dhamani* (? Rectal Arteries/ Veins/ Nerves/ Lymphatic Channels/Mucosa and Submucosa) because of the life style, especially like *Utkatkasana (excessive adaptation of deep squatting position)*, *Vishama Kathinasana* (Improper sitting on hard surfaces) and *Prishtayana (Excessive bicycle or bike riding, horse riding, camel and elephant riding)* etc.

This, leads to the *Khavaigunya* at the place of *Gudavali* (Mucosal Folds at Ano-rectal region). The *Sthana Samshraya (Nidus or Localization of the pathology)* of the *Dosha* takes place at the *Srotho Vaigunya* (Deformity, either Functional or Structural or Both, at the site of the Disease), which results into the vitiation of the *Twak (Skin), Mamsa (Muscle) and Meda (Fat and Loose Areolar Tissue) Dhatu (Tissues)*. The *Mamsa Dooshana* (Deformity in the Muscle and Mucosal Matrix), itself is indicative of the *Rakta Dooshana* (Blood Tissue abnormality) also, which is supported by the movement of *Dosha* along with the *Rakta (Blood)* towards the *Guda Bhaga* (Anal area) And even, the

Raktavasechana (Blood Letting) is one of the treatment modalities for *Arsha*.

when the person indulges in the *Vyadhi Hethu (Disease specific aetiology)* as well as *Vyanjaka hethu* (Precipitating aetiologies) like the washing of the *GudaBhaga* with *Sheethajala (extremely cold water), Upala (Cow dung Cakes), loshtra (type of stone), kashta (wooden piece)* and adopting postures like *Utkatakasana, Vishamasana* etc, and the habits like *Vegodeerana* (Forceful defecation) and *Pravahana* (Straining at Defecation) etc, this *Sthana Samshraya Avastha* (Stage of localization of the pathology) is converted into the *Vyaktavastha* (Stage of Clinical feature) very soon,

These *Mamsankura* (Piles or Sliding of the Anal Mucosa) become *Vyaktha (Visible)* at the *GudaBhaga* (Anal region) are called as Arsha (Piles). Arsha, may do the *Adhomargavarodha* (Obstruction to the faeces and flatus) to further vitiate all types of Vata dosha (*Apana, Prana,Udana, Vyana and Samana*) to worsen the condition, This leads into the manifestation of other systemic features like *Krishata* (Generalised Dark Discoloration/ Tanning/ Depigmentation), *Utsaha Hani* (Loss of enthusiasm), *Marma Peeda* (Pain at the Anus and other vital parts like Bladder, Flanks, Chest and at Umbilicus), *Kasa* (Cough), *Pipasa* (Excessive Thirst), *Shwasa* (Dyspnoea/ breathing Difficulty) and *Peenasa* (Running Nose/ Sinusitis).

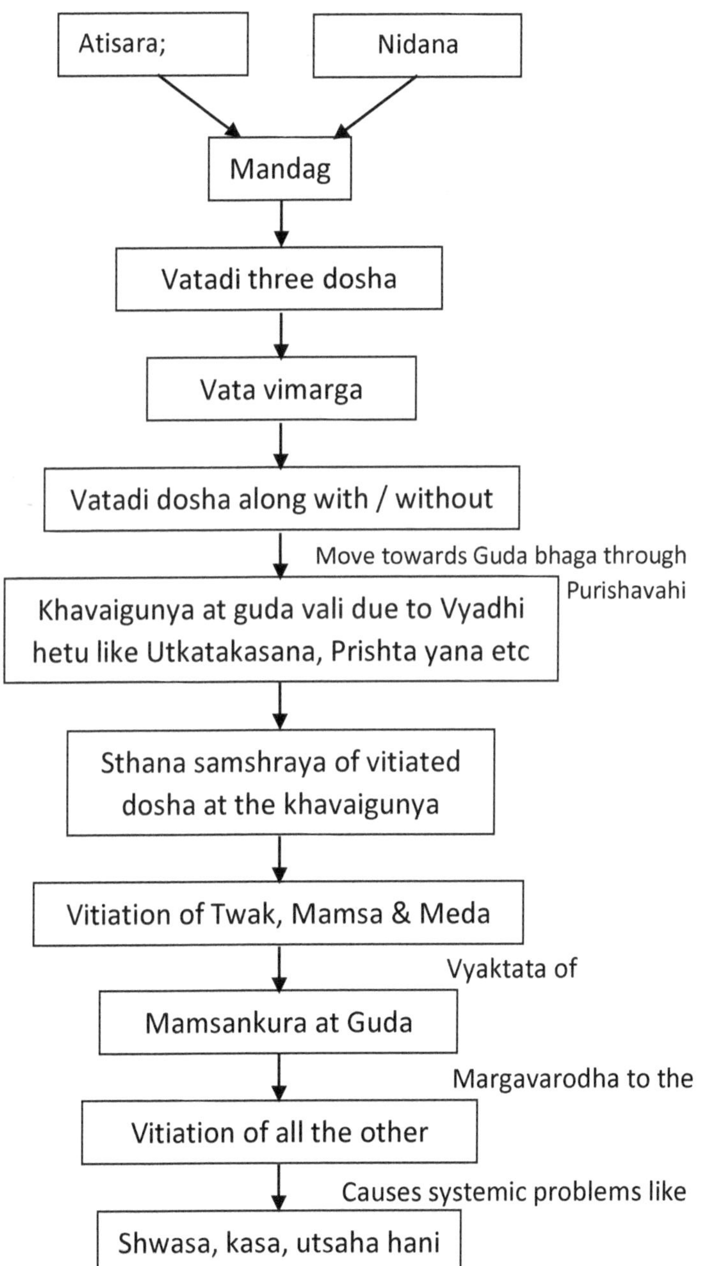
Atisara;
Nidana
Mandag
Vatadi three dosha
Vata vimarga
Vatadi dosha along with / without
Move towards Guda bhaga through
Purishavahi
Khavaigunya at guda vali due to Vyadhi
hetu like Utkatakasana, Prishta yana etc
Sthana samshraya of vitiated
dosha at the khavaigunya
Vitiation of Twak, Mamsa & Meda
Vyaktata of
Mamsankura at Guda
Margavarodha to the
Vitiation of all the other
Causes systemic problems like
Shwasa, kasa, utsaha hani

Vishishta Samprapti (Disease Specific Pathologenesis)[16]

The *Sahaja Arsha* (Congenital piles) having *Beejadosha* (genetic problem) as the causative factor, requires the *Vishishta Samprapti* to explain its manifestation as a disease. But the *Janmottara kalaja Arsha (Piles due to Acquired Causes)* with different dosha predominance, may involve the *Samprapti* (Pathology) as following;

Figure No.3: Vataja Arsha vishishta Samprapti

Indulgence in causative factors like shooka dhanya, kashaya, katu rasa, Ati Maithuna, Ati vyayama etc.

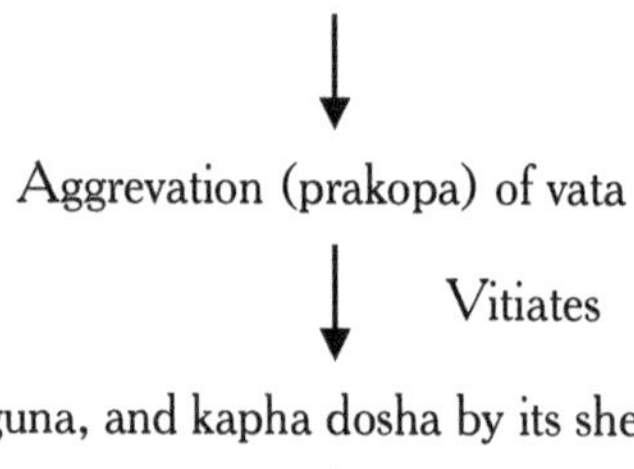

Aggrevation (prakopa) of vata

Vitiates

Pitta by laghu guna, and kapha dosha by its sheeta guna

All the Tridosha move towards the Guda bhaga through the pradhana dhamani

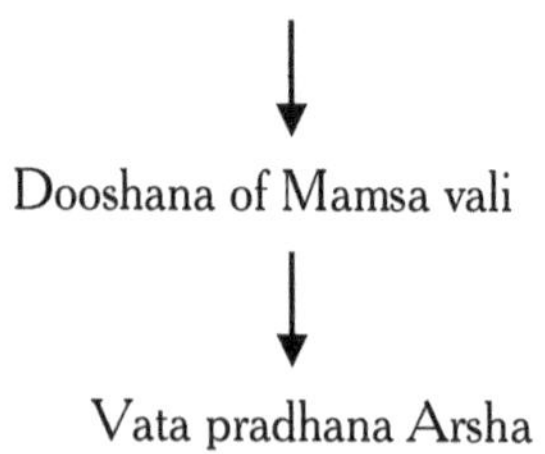

Dooshana of Mamsa vali

Vata pradhana Arsha

Figure No.4: Pittaja Arsha vishishta Samprapti

Indulgence in causative factors like Tila, Dadhi, Katu, Ushna, Kshara, Lavana, Ati Ushna Kala, Desha Sevana

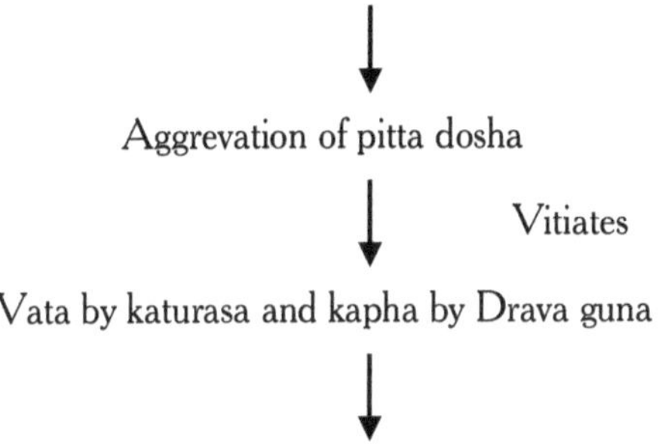

All the Tridosha move towards the Guda bhaga through the pradhana dhamani

Dooshana of mamsa vali

Pitta pradhana Arsha

Figure No.5: Khapaja Arsha vishishta Samprapti

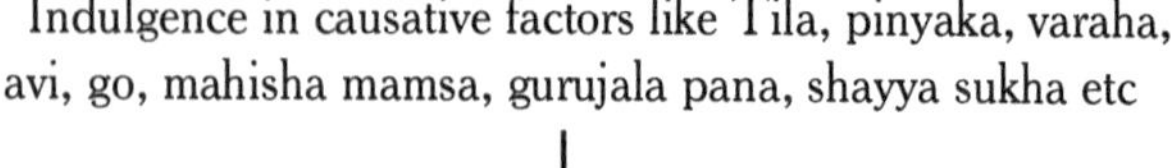

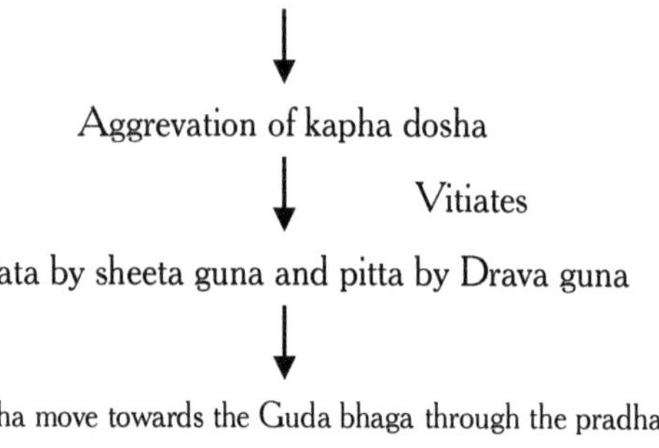

↓

Dooshana of mamsa vali

↓

Kapha pradhana Arsha

Samprapti Ghataka (Pathogenic Factors): The "*Chakravyuha*"(Hedge maze)

of the Samprapti can be broken down, if the knowledge about the Samprapti ghataka is clear. The Arsha roga is encircled with the ghataka as follows:

Vyadhi swabhava - chirakari
Udbhava Sthana - Amashaya and Pakvashaya
Vyaktasthana - Guda bhaga
Agni - Jathara Agni
Vata Pradhana Tridosha
Arsha
Adhishtana - Gudavali
Aama - Jathara Agni - mandya janya Ama - mamsa, raktha dhatvagni - mandya janya ama
Vyadhi swabhava - chirakari
Vyadhi swabhava - chirakari
Dooshya - twak, rakta, mamsa and meda
Srothas - mamsavaha, raktavaha & pureesha vaha
Sancharasthana, pureeshvahi dhamani
Srotodushti prakara - vimarga gamana, siragranti, sangha
Vyadhi swabhava - chirakari

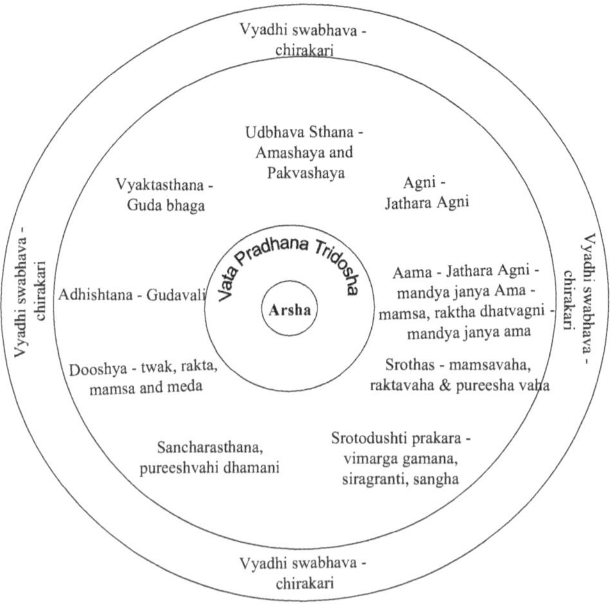

Samprapti (Pathogenesis)

Only knowing about the *Poorvaroopa (Prodromal Features)* and *Roopa (Clinical Features)*, will not be helpful to intervene in the *Samprapthi Vighatana (*Breaking the Pathological Process*)*. The treatment planned, without assessing the *Vyadhi Bala* (Intensity and progress of the Disease), fails to give the positive result in curing the disease. And, the *Vyadhi Bala* is assessed on the basis of the *Samprapti bheda (*Different Types and Modes of Pathogenesis of the disease*)*. Hence, the Arsha should be assessed on the basis of following *Samprapti bheda*.

1. ***Sankhya and Vidhi Samprapti:*** **(Classification of the Arsha)** The *Arsha*, is basically classified into two types depending upon its stage of occurrence like (1) *Sahaja* (Congenital) that is, which has occurred along with the birth and (2) *Janmottara kalaja* that is, which appears after the birth due to the practice of such regimen, which cause both the vitiation of *Dosha* (Humor) and

Dushya (Tissues), resulting into manifestation of Vyadhi (Disease), due to *Utpadaka hethu sevana* (Prime aetiologies)

The *Janmottara kalaja Arsha*, can be grossly classified into again two types, depending upon their nature of discharge or bleeding, which even indicate the predominance of the dosha involved in that particular Arsha. The Arsha, which do not bleed are termed as *ShushkArsha* (Dry Piles), predominant in *Vata* and *Kapha dosha*. Whereas those, which bleed are named as *Ardra Arsha*, predominant with the *Pitta Dosha* and *Raktha dushti* (vitiated Blood).

So, the reclassification can be made about the *Arsha* as of 6 types i.e., *Vataja, Pittaja, Khapaja, Sannipattaja, Raktaja and Sahaja*. The *Dvandvaja* type of *Arsha* need not be counted separately due to their *Prakruti Samasavayarabdhatva (Similarities)*. But, to be more specific in choosing the *Chikitsa* (Treatment), one can differentiate the Arsha as *Janmottara Kalaja* with *Vata, Pitta, Khapaja, Dvandvaja, Sannipataja, Shonitaja and Sahaja Arsha*.

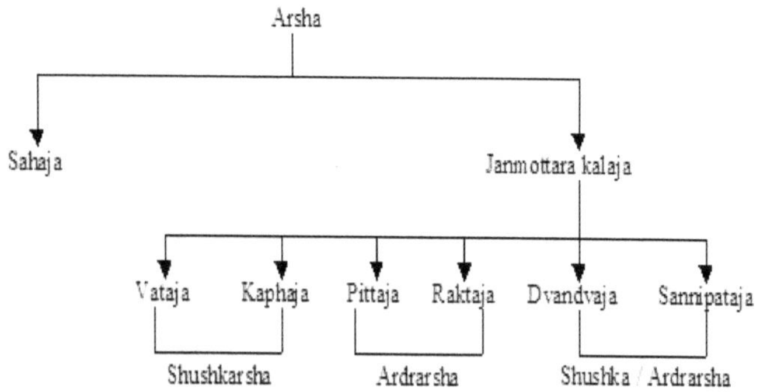

Figure No.7: Classification of Arsha

2. *Vikalpa Samprapti* (Permutation & Combination of Pathogenic Factors): The *Amshamshi kalpana* of *dosha* (Percentage wise evaluation of the pathogenic factors) involved, can be assessed in each *Arsha* separately, to treat the *Vyadhi* by the *Vipareet Chikitsa (Dosha, Vyadhi and Ubhaya Vipareeta)* (opposite of aetiologies treatments) following;

Vataja Arsha – The Nidana, that cause the vitiation of Vata dosha is by means of the Guna (Properties of materials) like Sheeta (Cold), Rooksha (Dryness) and Laghu (Lightness). Hence, the vitiated Vata along with its aggravated Guna, like Rooksha, Sheeta and Laghu (Gunathah Vikruti – Pathology by means of abnormal properties of homeostasis), takes the Vimargagamana (Karmataha Vikruti – Functional abnormality of the Physiology), moves upwards thus vitiating the Prana, Udana, Vyana and Samana (Types of Vata Dosha) along with the other two Dosha (The Pitta and Kapha). The vitiated Dosha with the predominance of the Vata dosha produces the Arsha with the signs like

- *Shyava Varna (rupatah vikruti of Vata)* {Brownie induration/ Thrombosed Piles}
- *Parusha (khara gunatha vikruti)* and {Rough surfaced piles}
- symptoms like the *Shula, Toda, Sphurana (karmatmaka vikruti)* etc. {Pain predominant like pricking, throbbing and severe discomfort}.

Pittaja Arsha: The Pittakara Nidana, (Aetiologies that aggravate Pitta Dosha) that are indulged in, will vitiate the Pitta by means of their Teekshna (piercing/penetrating), Ushna (Hot), Sara (Flowing), Amla (Sour Tasted), Visra (Offensive odour) and Drava Guna (Liquid property) to produce the Arsha with the signs like

- *Raktavarna (ragaha – roopataha vikruti)* {Red coloured mucosa over the piles}
- *Shonitha srava (drava gunataha vikruti) {Bleeding}*
- *Paka (teekshna gunataha vikruti) {Suppuration}*
- *Bhinnavarchah (sara gunataha vikruti) {Loose stools}*

- *Visra Gandhayukta Shonita Srava (gandataha dravyatmaka vikruti) {Bleeding is with offensive odor}*
- *symptoms like Daha (ushna gunataha vriddhi) {Burning Pain at the anal region}*
- *Kandu (karmatmaka vikruti) {Itching at the anal, due to the discharge}*

***Khapaja Arsha*:** These *Arsha* are presented with the signs like

- Shveta and Pandu Varna (roopataha dravyatmaka vikruti); {Pale coloured pile covering;both skin as well as mucosa}
- Shlakshna (shlakshna gunataha vriddhi); {Glistening Surface}
- Snigdha (snigdha gunataha vriddhi); {Moist and Unctuous}
- Sthabdha and supta suptata (sheeta gunataha vriddhi); {Less painful due to numbness sensation}
- Sthira shvayatu (guru gunataha vriddhi); {Prominent Swelling}
- Kandu (karmatmaka vikruti) {Prominent Pruritus- Anal Itching}
- Guru pichhila pichha and malasrava (dravyatmaka vikruti) {Mucous Mixed Stools}.

In the same way the Shonitaja (Blood vitiated Piles), Dvandvaja, Sannipataja and Sahaja Arsha should be assessed, before starting the treatment.

3. *Pradhanya Samprapti* (Predominant Dosha/ Pathogenic Factors) :Even though, the *Arsha* involves all the three *Dosha* in its manifestation, the *Vata dosha* is the main culprit in initiating the *Samprapti*. All sub variety of *Vata*, along with the *Pitta and Kapha Dosha* vitiate, the *Gudavali* to produce the *Arsha Roga*. Hence the *Arsha* can be termed as *Vata Pradhana Tridoshaja Vyadhi* (Disease produced due to the aggravation of all the three *Dosha)*.

But, the other *Dosha* may get upper hand and may become predominant in the further course of the disease, thus causing the

Pittolbana Arsha, *Kapholbana Arsha*, *Dvandvaja* and *Sannipataja Arsha* with the *Taratama Bhava* of the participating dosha.

4. Kala Samprapti (Influence of Age, Diurnal Cycle & Seasonal Changes) The *Sheeta kala* and *Desha (Cold Climate and Countries)*, aggravate the *Vatolbana Arsha*. In *Varsha Rutu (Rainy Season)*, the *Vata* which is already vitiated, further gets aggravated due to the *Ati Seetata* of the *kala (Extreme Coldness of the Season)*, may be because of *Mithya Yoga* (Winter super imposing over the Rainy season). This *Dosha* (Variation) may produce the *Vataja Arsha* or may aggravate the already existing *Vatolbana Arsha*.

Whereas, the *AtiYoga* of *Sheeta* (Extreme Coldness) in the *Hemanta Rutu* (Winter Season), further leads to the excessive *Sanchaya of Kapha dosha* (accumulation of Kapha) and results into the production of the *Kapholbana Arsha*.

The *Ati Sevana* of *Atapa* (Excessive exposure to Hot Sun), especially in the *Sharad Rutu* (Autumn), when the *Pitta* is in *Prakopavasta (Aggravated Stage)*, causes the *Pittolbana Arsha.*

5. *Bala Samprapti* (Assessment of the strength of The Patient and the Disease) The *Bala* (Strength) of the *Arsha Vyadhi* is to be assessed before starting the treatment. The *Vyadhi bala* indicates the *Sadhyasadhyatva* (Prognosis of the disease) as well as the treatment modality to be chosen for the *Arsha*. Hence, to assess the *Vyadhi bala*, one should calculate the *Balabala* (Proportion of the strength and weaknesses of the disease) by means of *Nidana (Aetiology)*, *Poorva Roopa (Prodromal Symptoms and Signs) and Roopa* (Clinical Manifestation) of the *Arsha.*

4

Poorva Roopa (Prodromal signs and symptoms) of Arsha

Poorvaroopa of Arsha:[17]

The *Poorvaroopa* (Prodromal Features) of the *Arsha* appear, when the vitiated *Dosha* acquire the *Sthana Sanshraya* (Localisation of Pathogenetic Factors) in the *Guda (Anal region)*, the *Moola (Site of Origin)* of the *Pureeshavaha Srotas (Colon)*, after causing the *Vikruti* (Vitiation/abnormality) of *Jatharagni (Digestive fire in the Gut)*. Hence, the *Lakshana* (Clinical Features) produced are:

Table No.4: Poorvarupa of Arsha

Koshtagata **(Gastrointestinal Tract)**	***Sarva shareeragata*** **(All over the Body)**	***Mala Pravrutti*** **(Defecation)**	***Guda gata*** **(Anal Area)**
Antra koojana (Bowel Gurgling), Kukshi Atopa (Flatulence in abdomen), Anne Arshadda (Anorexia), Vishtamba (Constipation), Amlika (Sour belching), Paridaha (Burning sensation), Udgara Bahulya (Excessive burping), Grahanidosha (IBS, Crohn's & Ulcerative colitis)	*Saktisadana (Weakness/ fatigue in Limbs) Karshya (Emaciation), Shwayathu (Oedema), Pandu (Anaemia), Kasa (Cough), Shwasa (Dyspnoea), Balahani (Lethargy), Bramaha (Vertigo), Tandra (Dizziness), Anidra (Insomnia), Indriya Dourbalya (Diminished efficiency of sense organs)*	*Alpa Vitkata* (Scanty Faeces)	*Guda parikartana (Cutting type of Pain in Anal Region)*

The Sthana Samshraya Avastha, requires both the Dosha-Dushya Ubhayashrita Chikitsa. The Dushya involved are mainly Twak, Mamsa, Meda and Rakta. Whereas, the Adhishtana of Vyadhi (Site of the disease) is Guda Valaya (Anal Mucosal Folds). Since, among the 4-fold treatment of the Arsha includes the Shastra, Kshara and Agni to be applied at the Guda Bhaga, one should know the Shareera of the Guda (Anatomy & Physiology of Anus and Rectum). Otherwise, the procedures may turn fatal as the Guda is one among the Sadhyomarma (Death causing Vital Part of the body, on injury).

Guda Shareera (Anatomy & Physiology of Anus and Rectum) [18]

Guda, which has got, the synonyms like *Apana* (Due to the action site of Apana Vata) and *Payu* (Due to its Motor function of Defecation) is the end or terminal part of the *Sthulantra* (Colon). Its situation in the *Gudasthi vivara* (Pelvic Cavity) is such that, it is related to the structures like *Basti* (Urinary Bladder), *Basti Shira* (Trigone of the Bladder), *Pourusha* (Prostate gland/Cervix) and *Vrushana* (Testicles & Scrotum). *Guda* one among the *Matruja Avayava* (Maternal Inheritance), is made up of three *Peshi* (Muscles) arranged in *Samudga (Circular)* type of *Sandhi (Conjoining)* pattern.[19]

The total length of the *Guda* measures about 4 ½ *Anguli* (Anguli is scale of length, specific to each individual, as of length of crease of interphalangeal joint of finger) of his, and the diameter measures about four *Angula*. The whole length from the terminal part of *Sthulantra* (Large Colon) till the *Gudoushta* (Anal verge), is having the colour of the tongue of elephant (Pink). The main function of the *Payu*, which is one of the *Karmendriya* (Motor organ), is well understood as the *Pureesha nishkramana* (Excretion of Faeces), which is possible because of the presence of the, three *Vali* (Circular Anal Folds) in it.

The first *Vali* is situated one *Anguli* away from the *Gudoshta (Anal Verge)*, which is situated one and half *Yava (Grain of Barley-Hordeum vulgare)* length from the *Romantha Bhaga* (Anal verge with hairs). This *Vali* is named as *Samvarani*. *Visarjini* is the second *Vali* from outside inwards, situated at a distance of one and half *Anguli* from the *Samvarani*. Whereas, *Pravahini*, the third *Vali* is situated at the same distance i.e., one and half *Anguli* from the *Visarjini Vali*. These *Valie* are circular as of the *Shankanabhi* (Internal stem of Conch Shell), with elevation of about one *Anguli*.

As the *Guda* is the *Moola* of the *Pureeshavaha Srotas (Channel for the faeces),* along with the *Pakwashaya (Large Colon and Rectum)*, does take the role in the formation and excretion of the *Pureesha* (Faeces). *Guda*, which is divided into two parts as *Uttara Guda* (Proximal part of the Rectum) and *Adhara Guda* (Distal Part of Rectum including the Anal canal), finds its main function as the storage and excretion of the *Pureesha* (Stools) The *Uttara Guda* is the place for the storage of the *Pureesha*, whereas, the *Adhara Guda*, does the *Pureesha nishkramana kriya* (Defecation). The whole act of *Pureesha Nishkramana* is done by the *Gudavali* with the initiation by the *Pureeshavahi Dhamani (Rectal Vessels and Nerves)*, which are, two among the *Adhogami Dhamani (Downward Going Vessels)*.

The inner most *Vali* i.e., *Pravahini* pushes the *Pureesha* downwards towards the *Visarjini*. The *Visarjini Vali*, becomes distended after receiving the *Pureesha*, pushes the *Pureesha* outside of the body through the *Bahirmukha Srothas* (Outward leading channel of the body) i.e., *Guda* (Anus). The *Pureesha* is cut into segments by the *Samvaranivali* once, the *Pureesha* passes past that *Vali* to facilitate the defaecation and closes the *Gudamarga (Anal orifice)*.

Because of its complex structure, the *Guda*, one among the *Dasha Pranayathana* (Ten Sites of Life Energy) and *Sadhyomarma* (Death causing Vital Part, on Injury) is truly the *Moola* (Root) of the *Shareera (Body)*.

Figure No. 8: Guda Shareera

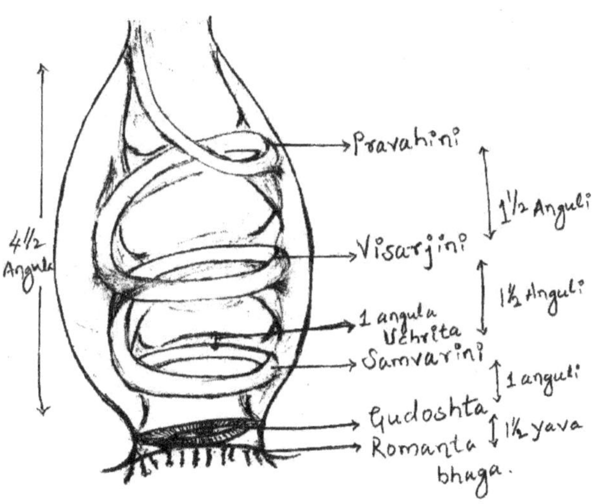

5

Roopa (Clinical Features / Signs and Symptoms) of Arsha

Once the *Samprapti* enters into the fifth *Kriyakala (Stages of Pathology)* i.e., *Vyaktavasta* (Stage of Clinical Presentation) from the *Sthana samshraya (poorva roopavasta)* (Stage of Pre-Clinical stage), it produces the *Vishishta Roopa (Specific clinical feature)* of the *Arsha Vyadhi* as *Mamsankura* (Fleshy projections) at the *Guda Pradesha* (Anal Region)

The features of these *Mamsankura*, vary according to the predominance of the *Dosha* in the manifestation of the disease, along with the other *Samanya Roopa* (General Clinical Feature) of the Humoral Constitution.

Table No.5: Vataja Arsha[20]

Lakshana of Arshankura	***Sarvangagata lakshana***	***Upadrava***	***Mala pravrutti***
Appearance – *Soochivat teekshnagra, resembles kadamba pushpa; tundikeri;* *bimbi; karakandu;* *kharjura; karpasi phala;* Colour: *Shyava, aruna* On touch – *Shuska, parusha, kathina, khara, sputitha.*	Pain in *kati, prishta, parshva, medhra, Guda and nabhi.* *Akshepa, toda,* *sphurana, chimachimayana, samhArsha,* Colour – *Shyava of twak, netra, nakha, vit, mootra, vaktra*	*Gulma, ashtheela, pleeha, udara*	*Shushka, alpa, vitkata of shyava varna along with pain.*

Table No.6: Pittaja Arsha[21]

Lakshana of Arshankura	***Sarvangagata lakshana***	***Upadrava***	***Mala pravrutti***
Appearance –Resembles *Jalouka vaktra* Colour: *As of neela, peetavabhasa, yakrut khanda, shukajeevha, krishna* On touch – *Mrudhu, shithila, aspArshasaha* Discharge – *Atikleda and dhurgandha yukta rakta* Course – *Leads into paka*	*Daha, kandu, shoola, nistoda in Guda.*	*Jwara, daha, pipasa, moorcha, tamaka, samhoha, bhojana dwesha,* Colour – *Peeta, twak, netra, nakha, vit, mootra, vaktra*	*Sarakta, sadaha, mala praVrutti.*

Table No.7: Khapaja Arsha[22]

Lakshana of Arshankura	***Sarvangagata lakshana***	***Upadrava***	***Mala pravrutti***
Appearance – Resembles *Kareera beeja, panasa beeja, gostana, mahamoolayukta* Colour: *Pandu varna* On touch – *Mrudu, shlakshna, guru, sthira, pichhila, spArsha priya.* Discharge – *Pichhila srava* Course – *Kandu at the Guda Bhaga*	*Sthabdata, staiMityaat the Arshankura.* *Guru, pichhila, shwetha, mootra*	*Pravahika, anaha in vankshana, parikartika, hrullasa, nishtivika, kasa, arochaka, pratishyaya, gourava, chardi, mootra kruchra, shosha, shotha, pandu, sheeta jwara, ashmari, sharkara etc.* Colour – *Shukla twak, netra, nakha, vit, mootra, vaktra*	*Guru, pichhila, shweta Kapha yukta mala in large quantity that resembles mamsa dhavita jala.*

Table No. 8: *RaktArsha*[23]

Presents in two different ways according to the predominance of the *Dosha* i.e.,

- Vatanubandhi RaktArsha (Vata associated Bleeding Piles)
- Kaphanubandhi RaktArsha (Kapha associated Bleeding piles)

Lakshana of Arshankura	***Sarvangagata lakshana***	***Upadrava***	***Mala praVrutti***
Appearance – Resembles *Nyagrodhapraroha, vidruma, gunjaphala, and other features of Pittaja Arshankura.* Discharge – *Raktasrava* Course – *Leads into paka*	*Vatanubandhi: - Avarodha of adhoVata, pain in kati, uru and Guda; dourbalya*	*Akshepaka, raktaPitta, jwara, trishna, agnisada, arochaka, kamala, pandu, shoola in Guda, kandu all over the body, kotha, pidaka, shotha. Vibandha to mootra pureesha and Vata. Bala, utsaha, varna and vojohani.*	*Vatanubandhi – Shyava, aruna varnayukta khatina, rooksha mixed with arunavarna yukta phenila rakta.* *Kaphanubandhi: Shithila, guru, snigdha, sheetala, shweta and peetha coloured mixed with ghana pichhila tantuyukta rakta.*

Sannipataja Arsha – Presents with the combination of all the three *dosha* with *prakruti sama- samavaya lakshana.*

Sahaja Arsha – *Arsha* that occurs as the *Adi bala pravrutta Vyadhi*, bears the features like *Parusha* (Rough surfaced), *Pandu Varna Yukta Arshankura* (Pale coloured mucosa covered interno-external piles). Which, may be small, may be big, may be elongated or short; may be round ball like or may be with irregularly spread base; they may be protruded outside or remain inside. These *Sahaja Arsha* (Congenital) present as per the *Anubandha of the Dosha (Association of either of any three humors, or two of the humors or one of the humor).*

Upadrava – The general features of the *sahaja Arshayukta* person, are indicative of gross impairment in the *agni* and other *chayapachaya (Metabolism)* of the body like - emaciated (*atikrusha)*, pigmentation in the skin *(vaivarna)*, weak (*sudurbala)* and *bhinnaswara* etc.

Fig: No. 9: Vata kaphaja arsha
External Piles

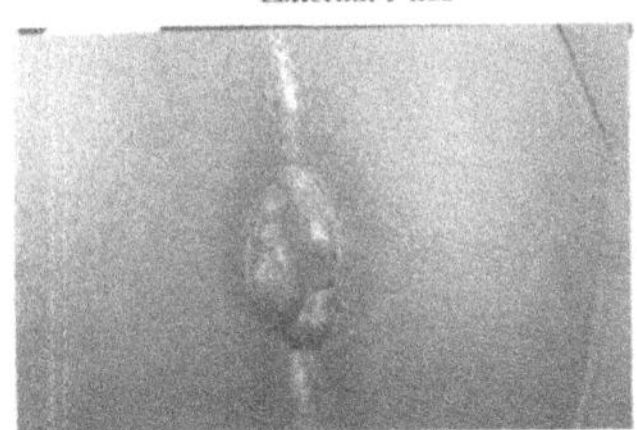

Fig: No. 10: Vataja arsha
External Piles

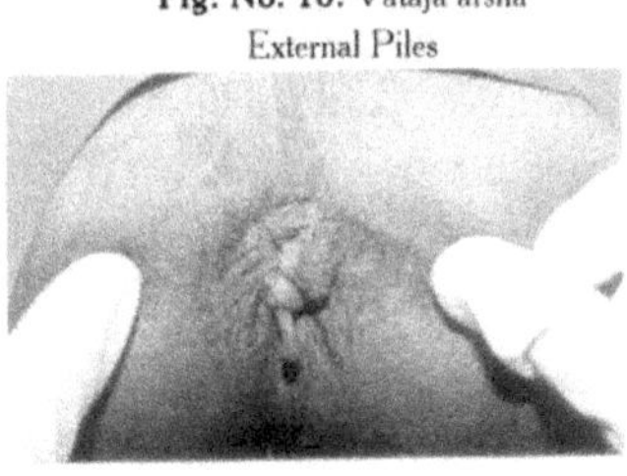

Fig: No.11: Dushta rakta sanchita arshankura
Thrombsed External piles

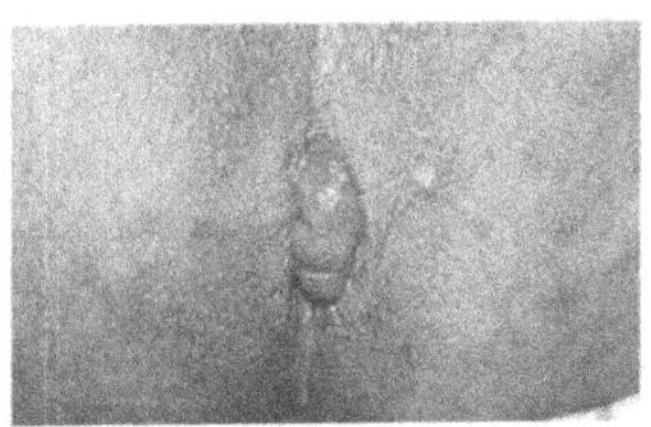

Fig: No.12: Kaphaja arshankura
Interno- External Piles

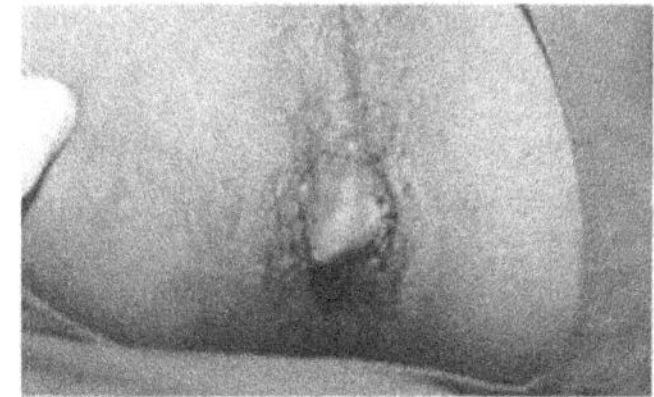

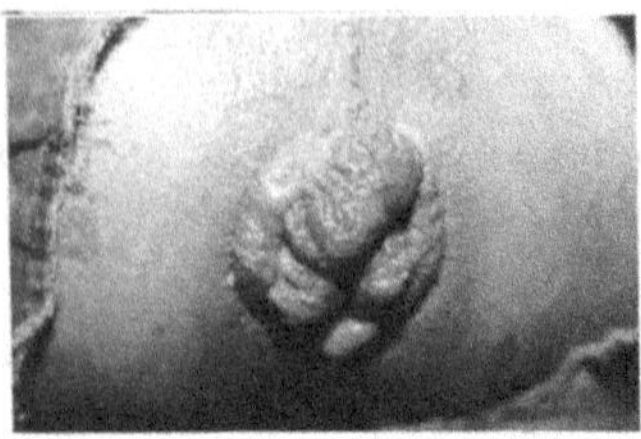

Fig: No. 13: *Pittaja Arshankura*
Prolapsed Internal piles 4th Degree

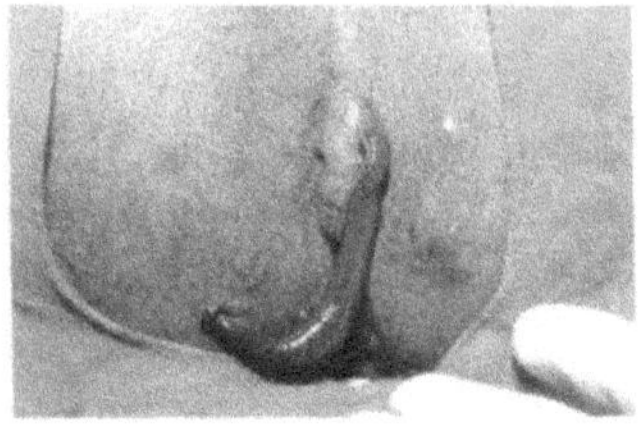

Fig: No. 14: *Raktavasechana* in *Arshankura*
Leech application in External.Thrombosed Piles

He passes the stools sometimes hard (*Vibadda*) or loose (*Mukta*); *Pakwa (Suppuration)* or *Ama (Metabolic Toxins)*; *Shushka (Dry)* and *Bhinna (inconsistent)*. Which is either white (*Shweta*), *Pandu (Pale)*, *Harita (Greenish yellow)*, *Peeta (Yellow)*, *Rakta* or *Arunavarnayukta (Red/Brick red colour)*. Stools, may be *Tanu* (Thin consistency) or *Sandra* (Thick) in consistency, mixed with *Pichhila* (Unctuous) and *Kunapa Gandhayukta Ama (Foul smelling Mucous discharge)*.

He experiences pain (*Parikartana*) at *Nabhi (Umbilicus)*, *Basti (Bladder)*, *Vankshana (Iliac fossae)*, *Guda (Anus)*, *Parshwa (Lumbar regions) and Sarva Asthi (All bony parts)*. There may be stiffness in *Parshwa (Lumbar region)*, *Kukshi (Abdomen & Pelvis)*, *Basthi (Bladder)*, *Hridaya Pradesha (Cardiac region)*, *Prishta (Lumbar region) and Trika (Sacral part)*. He is always troubled with *Pravahika* (Amoebic colitis), Pariharsha (Horripulation), Prameha (Diabetis Mellitus), *Vishtamba* (Constipation), *Antrakujana* (Bowel Gargling Sound), Udavarta (Flatulence), Upalepa of Hridaya and Indriya (Dizziness & heaviness at Heart And Senses), *Tiktamlodgara* (Sour belching), *Kasa (Cough)*, *Shwasa* (Dyspnoea), *Tamaka* (Bronchial Asthma), *Trishna* (Thirst), *Hrullasa* (Nausea), *Chardi* (Vomiting), *Arochaka* (Tastelessness), *Avipaka* (Indigestion), *Peenasa* (Running Nose), *Shwayatu* (Oedema), *Timira* (Cataract), *Shira Shoola (Headache)*, *Karnaroga* (Ear Disease), *Shotha in pani, pada, vadana and akshikoota* (Oedema in hand, feet, face and peri orbital area) and *Angamarda* (Malaise).

Since he is having *Durbalagni (Loss of Appetite)*, *Alpashukra (Azoospermia/Oligospermia)* and *Durbala Shareera (Weaker physics)* always remains frustrated, which will be expressed through the *Krodha (Anger)* and *Dukha (Grief)*.

6

Upashaya (Pacifying factors) - *Anupashaya* (Aggravating Factors):

Vatolbana Arsha – The measures like foodstuffs or physical activities or seasonal changes, which are *Snigdha* (Unctuous) and *Ushna* (Warm) in nature, act as the *Upashaya (pacifying)* for the *Vatolbana Arsha* (Vata predominant piles), because of opposite properties.

Pittolbana Arsha – Those regimens, which are *Sheeta* (Cold) in the *Guna* (Properties), *Veerya* (Potency of the drugs and food) and *Sparsha* (Touch), will reduce the intensity of *Pittolbana Arsha* (Pitta Predominant Piles).

Kapholbana Arsha: - The factors that are *Rooksha* (Dry) and *Ushna* (Hot) in *Guna*, *Veerya* and *Sparsha* will act to reduce the intensity of *Kapholbana Arsha* (Kapha Predominant piles).

Anupashaya: - Similar properties, as of the properties of the *Dosha*, will aggravate the *Dosha*, to cause the aggravation in the intensity of the disease. Thus, referred as *Anupashaya* (Aggravating Factors).

Special condition:[24]

When the *Arshankura* is accumulated with *Dushta Rakta* (Vitiated Blood), all the measures, let they may be, *Sheeta* (Cold) or *Ushna* (Hot) and *Snigdha* (Unctuous) or *Rooksha* (Dry), will not subside the disease and pain. Thus, if these *Upashaya* (Pacifying Factors) of the *Ekadoshaja Arsha* (Single Doshik Predominance) fail, then one should consider the condition is as because of the *Dushta Rakta* (Vitiated Blood), and should subject for the *Rakta Visravana* (Blood Letting Therapy), either by

Shastra (Incisions by surgical knife), *Soochi* (Needle/Scalp vein set needle/Intravenous Canula) or *Jalouka* (Leech Application), as per the involvement of the dosha, that will subside the condition.

7

Sadhyasadhyatwa (Prognosis of The Disease):[25]

The prognosis of the *Arsha* can be assessed on the basis of the following criterions.

1. Position of *Arshankura* (Pile Mass) in the *Gudavali (Anal Mucosal Folds)*
2. Duration of the *Vyadhi (Disease)*
3. Involvement of the *Dosha (Humor)*
4. Presentation of the disease with / without the association of *Upadrava (Complications)*

Table No.9: *Sadhya-Asadhyatva (Prognosis of the Disease)*

Criteria for prognosis	***Sukha sadhya (Easily Curable)***	***Krichhra sadhya (Cured with Difficulty)***	***Yapya (Cannot be Cured completely but Manageable/Controlled)***	***Asadhya (Incurable)***
Position of *Arshankura* in the *Gudavali*.	*Bahyavali ashrita* (*Samvarani*)	*Dviteeyavali ashrita (Visarjini)*	*Antarvali ashrita (Pravahini)*	*Antarvali ashrita (Pravahini)*
Duration of the *Vyadhi*	*Chirotpanna (of short duration)*	*Pari samvatsarani (ateeta)* (Of more than one year)	---	*Sahaja*
Involvement of the *Dosha*	*Ekadoshaja*	*Dwandwaja*	*Tridoshaja*	---
Upadravayukta	---	---	*Shesha ayu* and presence of *chatushpada* and *deepta kayagni*	*Shotha* in *hasta, pada* etc, *nishesha ayu*.

8

Chikitsa Upakrama of Arsha (Treatment Modalities)

The *Arsha* is such a severe disease, which has got different modalities of the treatment. Each stage through which it passes, has got the unique treatment designed specifically to treat the cause to have the effect as a disease-free status.

The total four -fold treatment like *Bheshaja, Shastra, Kshara and Agni* have got their intervention, depending on the intensity of the disease.[26] The *Bheshaja chikitsa* is employed when *Arsha* are *Adrushya* (invisible) or even in the *Drushya Arsha* (Visible) of *Alpakala* (of less duration) and associated with the less intensive features. Further, the *Arsha rogi* (Piles Patient), who requires *Bheshaja chikitsa*, if is passing the *Baddhamala* (hard stools), then the treatment is planned on the line of treatment of *Udavarta* (Treatment advocated for the Flatulence and its complications). If he is passing the *Bhinnavarcha* (loose stools), then the treatment is planned as per the line of treatment of *Vataja Atisara (Frothy Diarrhoea)*, especially in case of *Vatolbana Arsha*. If the bleeding is associated in the *Arsha rogi*, then it should be taken care by the treatment either as of *Pittaja Atisara (Bloody Diarrhoea)* or as of *RaktaPitta* (Bleeding Diseases like Haemophilia/ Epistaxis/Bleeding Diathesis).[27]

The *ShushkArsha* (Dry Piles/ Non- Bleeding Piles/ Non - Discharging Piles), which includes both the *Vatolbana* and the *Kapholbana Arsha*, when becomes visible, should be treated with both, the *Bahiparimarjana* (External Application of Medicament or Para-surgical Procedures or Surgery) and *Antahaparimarjana chikitsa (Internal Medications either Oral or Rectal route)*. *Bahiparimarjana chikitsa* (Integrated, both External and Internal Measures) includes *teekshna pralepa* (Stringent Medicament

Applications), *Swedana (Sudation)*, *Avagaha sweda* (Hot Sitz Bath) and *Parisheka* (Showering of Medicated Decoctions, Oils, Ghee etc). Antahaparimarjana chikitsa is planned with the *Shodhana (Purification or Detoxification Therapies, popularly known as Panchakrma)* and *Shamana* (Pacifying Medications) with various combinations of the drugs.

Ardra Arsha (Bleeding or Discharging Piles) like *Pittolbana* and *RaktArsha* (Haemorrhoids), should be treated with the *Bheshaja* (Medicines) used in *RaktaPitta* (Bleeding Diathesis), once all the *Dushta Shonita* (Vitiated Blood) is drained out.

Once the *Arsha* grows, beyond the stage of *Bheshaja Sadhya Chikitsa (Medical or Conservative Management)*, and becomes *Drushya* (Visible outside the Anal Verge), then the *Shastrakarma* (Surgical Excision), *Ksharakarma* (Chemical Cauterization) or *Agnikarma* (Thermal Cauterization or Laser Therapy) will be employed as per the indication.

Bheshaja Chikitsa (Medicinal Management):

The *Dravyabhoota chikitsa (Treatment with the Materials like Tablets, Powders, Decoction, Capsules, Injectables, Local Applications of Ointments/Solutions/hot & cold fomentations etc)* with *Bheshaja (Medicine)* for *Arsha rogi* (Piles Patient) depends upon the following criteria.

- *Drushya (Visible outside the Anal Verge, means either external piles or Prolapsed internal piles)* or *Adrushya Arshankura (Internal First-Degree Piles, that Does not Prolapse outside the Anal Verge)*
- *Baddhamala (Constipated and/or Hard Stools)* or *Bhinnavarcha (Loose and Inconsistent Stools)*
- Shushka (Nonbleeding/ non discharging) and *Ardra Arsha* (Bleeding/Discharging)

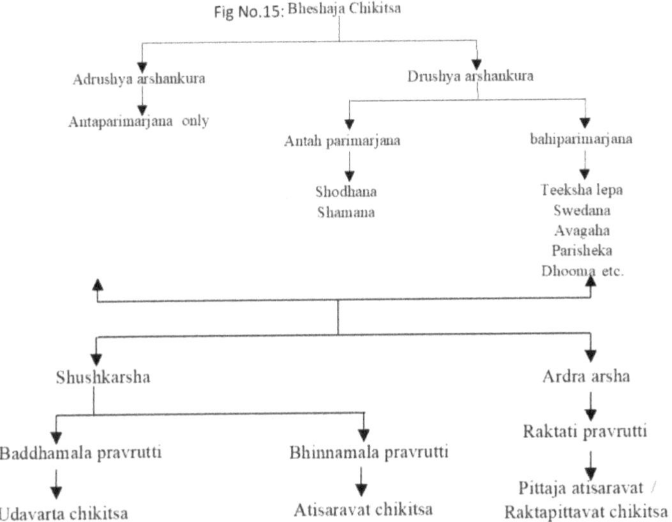

Indication for Bheshaja chikitsa

- *Adrushya Arshankura* (First Degree Piles)
- *Drushya Arshankura* (Second Degree Onwards) of

Achirakalajata (of less duration)

Alpadoshayukta (of less intense dosha)

Alpa lakshana (with a smaller number of features)

Alpaupadrava (with a smaller number of complications)

<u>Chikitsa of Adrushya Arshankura</u> – This is always done with *Antaparimarjana chikitsa*, which includes both *Shamana and Shodhana* as per the need, depending upon the *Doshabala* (Extent of vitiation of the Dosha).

<u>Shodhana (Purification or Detoxification Therapies):</u> Shodhana, by means of Vamana (Emesis), Virechana (Purgation) and Asthapana (Medicated Enema) therapy, in case of Pravridda Dosha (Highly aggravated Dosha) is adopted to drain out the Dosha to cure the condition, which will not allow the disease to reoccur.

The *Vamana* can be applied in the *Vataja Arsha*, associated with *Kapha Prakopa lakshana (Features of Kapha Dosha Aggravation)* like *Kapha Praseka (Excessive Salivation)* and in the *Kapha Pradhana Arsha*, before the administration of *Shamanoushadhi* (Pacifying Medications).

The *Snaihika Virechana* (Purgation with Unctuous Medicines) is employed, with the help of *Eranda Taila* (Caster oil) mixed with *Triphala Kwatha*, to drain out the *Pitta & Shleshma (Kapha)* and to regularise the movement of *Vata*, by initiating the *Vatanulomana* in the patients with the *Vit Vibandha* (Impacted Stools) and *Pravridda Dosha (Aggravated Dosha)*.[29]

The application of *Basti* (Medicated Enema), either *Asthapana* (Decoction Enema) orAanuvasana (Oil/Ghee/Fat/Marrow used Enema), is dependent upon the *Lakshana* of the *Arshankura*. Thus, the *Basti* finds its indication mainly in the *Drushya Arshankura*, even though it can be used in the *Adrushya* (Non prolapsing) *Arshankur.*

Aoushadhi Yoga for Adrushya Arsha -[30]

- *Guda + Haritaki* – early in the morning
- *Gomutra Siddha Haritaki + Kshoudra* – in *Gadavit* and *Mandagni* - early in the morning
- *Ballataka Choorna + Takra* – in *KaphaVataja (shushkArsha)*
- *Chitraka Chdoorana Siddha Ksheera* – in *Kapha Pradhana Arsha*, with the *Mandagni and Baddhamala.*
- *Shrungavera+Punarnava+ChitrakaKashaya Siddha Ksheera– KaphaVatanubandi RaktArsha.*
- *Kutaja Moola Twak Phanita – in Kapha Pittanubandha RaktArsha.*

Chikitsa of Drushya Arshankura – *Drushya Arshankura*, which do not bleed are usually *Kapholbana* and Vatolbana Arsha, and are considered as the *ShushkArsha*. Whereas, the *Pittolbana and Shonitaja Arsha*, which bleed are termed as *Aardra Arsha*. The features of the *Arshankura* itself, give the picture of the *Dosha Pradhanata* and the shushka or ardra Arsha.

Chikitsa of Shushka Arsha – Among the *Shodhana* therapies, other than the *Vamana* and *Virechana*, which are mentioned earlier, the *Asthapana* and *Anuvashana basthi* find their indication in *ShushkArsha*.

Basti therapy in Arsha – *Nirooha Basti (Decoction Enema)* with *Dashamoola Kashaya*, *Godugdha* and *Gomutra* is useful in *ShushkArsha* associated with the *Udavarta* and *VilomaVata* (Opposite moving *Vata*).[31]

Eranda Mooladi Niruha Basti can be used in the *Vatolbana Arsha*, associated with the *Kapha* and *Vit Avarana* {*Vata* Obstructed by the Loaded Rectum (impacted stools)} to the *ApanaVata*.[32] Whereas, the *Kapholbana Arsha rogi*, can be administered with *Teekshna Basti (Stringent Enema)*.[33]

The combination of *Panchamoola Kwatha*, *Ksheera* and *Gomutra*, along with *Sneha, Lavana and Kalka of Madanaphala, Bilwa* etc is used as *Niruha Basti* in the *ShushkArsha rogi*, suffering with *Udavarta* and *Vatavilomagati*.

When the patient suffers with the *Udavarta* and *Shoola* (Pain in Abdomen) due to the *Vilomagati of Vata*, that is aggravated due to the excessive *Virukshana* (Dryness), should be treated with *Anuvasana Basti*.[34]

Pippalyadi Anuvasana Basti has got good effect in relieving, the *Udavarta* and *Shoola* by inducing *Snigdhata* in the *Koshta* (Gastro intestinal Tract) and doing *Vatanulomana*. The *Anuvasana basti* is mainly used in *Vatolbana Arsha*, among the *ShushkArsha*. If, the *Anuvasana basti* is used in the *Avruta Vatajanya Arsha*, that may cause *Snigdhta* in the *Arsha* and *Adhmana*. So, the *Anuvasana* is used, only in the *Shuddha Vata* state to avoid the production of *Upadrava* (Complications).

Chikitsa of baddhamalayukta Arsha rogi **(Constipated or Hard Stool)**– The *Shamana Aoushadhi (Pacifying Medicines)*, thus administered in case of *Arsha Rogi* passing *Baddhamala*, should remove the *Vibaddhata*, should do the *Vatanulomana* and *Agnideepana (Increases the Metabolic rate)*. For this reason, the *Udavarta* like *Chikitsa*, should be followed by using different drugs, in different forms as following

1. *Varuni* + *Sneha* + *Saktu* + *Lavana*.
2. *Karanjapatra Yamaka* before food.
3. *Ghrita like Palashadi, Panchakoladi,* Changeryadi, *Pippalyadi* etc before food.
4. *Gomutra Siddha Haritaki* in the number of two per day to get rid of *ShushkArsha* with *BaddhaVitkata*.
5. *Kshara* like *Kalyanaka Kshara* and *Mahakshara* along with either *Guda* or *Ghrita* can be taken before food to brighten up the *Agni*, thus removing the *Malabaddhata* by means of *Vatanulomana*.

Chikitsa of Bhinnamalayukta Arsha rogi **(Loose or inconsistent Stool)**– Patients of *Shushka Arsha* passing loose stools, should be treated as of *Atisara* (diarrhoea). So, the drugs which will be used, are administered with the *Anupana of Takra* (Along with the Butter Milk) to get better result.

Takra praYoga (Usage of Butter Milk):

The *Takra*, which is the ultimate *Bheshaja* in the *Vataja and Khapaja Arsha*, is used along with the *Sneha* (Unctuousness inducing substances) in case of *Vataja Arsha* and without *Sneha* in case of *Kapholbana Arsha*. It can be used for longer period, with the combination of other drugs that are *Agni Deepaka* and *Vatanulomaka*. Some of the combinations are as follows.

1. *Haritaki + Takra*
2. *Triphala Choorna + Takra*
3. *Chitraka + Hapusha + Hingu +Takra*
4. *Panchakola Choorna + Takra*
5. *Takrarishta*
6. *Takravaleha*

The *Takra*, either *Rooksha* or *Ardhoddhruta Snehayukta* (half part of *Sneha*) or *Anuddhruta Ghrita* (having whole part of *Sneha*), is used as per the need after assessing the percentage of the *Dosha* involved. The quantity of daily intake of *Takra*, should be gradually increased along with the reduction in the quantity of solid food, for the duration of one month, so that, at the end of the month, patient will be kept only on the *Takra*, till the disease is cured. Once the relief from the complaint is achieved, the quantity of the *Takra* is reduced gradually along with the gradual increase in the intake of the food with in the period of one month. By this, the *ShushkArsha* associated with *Bhinnavarcha*, is cured.

Bahiparimarjana chikitsa for shushkArsha (External Applications)

When, the *ShushkArsha* is prolapsed outside and is associated with the *Lakshana* like *Guruta (Heaviness), Kandu (Itching), Shopha (Oedema), Shoola (Pain)* and it could not be treated with the *Shastra, Kshara or Agni*, because of some technical problem (Patient unfit for the surgery), then one should use the *Bahiparimarjana Chikitsa (External Measures)* as *Lepa (Smearing of medicated Pastes), Pindasweda (Type of Sudation), Dravasweda (Sudation with Hot Liquids), Dhoopana (Fumigation of Pile mass & The Patient with medicines)* etc. By, the application of *Bahiparimarjana chikitsa*, the *Arshankura* may fall off or the accumulated *Dooshita Rakta* may be drained out.[35]

Lepa Yoga (Paste formulations) –

- *Kaseesadi taila*
- *Snuhi ksheera + haridra choorna*
    - *Kushta + shirisha beeja + pippali + saindhava + Guda + arka ksheera +sudha ksheera + triphala*
- *Pippalyadi lepa*
- *Arshoghna lepa*
- *Sooranadi lepa*
- *Arka ksheeradi lepa*

Pindasweda and Avagahasweda (Sudation with a Ball of different material and Sitz Bath)

The application of the *Lepa* (Application of Paste), should be followed with the *Pindasweda* (Sudation with a Ball of different Materials) and *Avagahasweda* (Sudation with Sitz Bath). Usually, the *Pindasweda* with the *Pindi* (Ball) prepared by either *Yava (Barley), Kulattha, Masha, Gomaya (Cow dung), Khara Shakrut (Donkey's Excreta), Ashwa Shakrut (Horse Excreta) or Tila Kalka* (Paste of Seasum Seeds) should be applied to the *Arshankura* after the *Abhyanga* (Massage) by the *Siddha Taila* (Medicated Oil).

When the patient complains of the *Shoola* (Pain), then the *Abhyanga* (Massages) of the *Arshankura* (Piles) should be followed by, the *Avagahasweda* with the *Kwatha* (Decoction) of either *Moolaka, Triphala, Arka, Venu, Varuna* etc. Even *Ushnajala* (Warm water) in *Sheeta Kala* (Cold Climate) and *Sheetajala (Cold Water)* in *Ushna Kala* (Hot Climate) can be used.

Dhoopana (Fumigation):

Dhoopana with bark of *Arka Moola* or *Shamee Patra*, should be applied after the *Abhyanga* (Massage) of the *Arshankura* (Piles), to subside the pain.

If all these measures fail to give relief to the patient, from the pain, then the accumulated impure blood is drained out by proper measures.

Rakta mokshana (Blood Letting Therapy)

The *ShushkArsha* (Non-Bleeding or Non-Discharging Piles), when they are associated with accumulation of vitiated blood, will produce severe pain which is not relieved either by *Sheeta* (Cold Measures) or *Ushna* (Hot Measures) and *Snigdha* (Unctuousness) or *Rooksha* (Dryness) measures. This requires intervention with *Rakta Mokshana*, by using, either *Jalouka (Leech), Shastra (Surgical incision or Venesection) or Soochi (Scalp vein set or big bore needle)* as per the need, to drain out the *Dushta Rakta (Vitiated or Toxic Blood)* to get the relief.

Chikitsa of Ardra Arsha (Treatment of Bleeding or Discharging Piles)

Pittaja and *Shonitaja Arsha* give rise to *Raktasrava* (Bleeding), to appear as ardra *Arsha*. The following principles should be followed as per the condition to treat the *Ardra Arsha.*[36,37]

Table No.10: Summarised Chikitsa Upakrama of RaktArsha (Treatment modalities of Bleeding Piles/ Haemorrhoids)

Condition	Principles
Vatanubandhi RaktArsha	*Snehapana, Abhyanga and Anuvasana; Snigdha Sheeta Annapana*
Kaphanubandhi raktArsha	*Rooksha and Sheeta Ahara, Aoushadhi and Vihara*
Pitta Sleshmanubandhi RaktArsha	*Pachana, Deepana, Vamana and Virechana; allowing the Raktasrava to achieve Langhana effect*
Vata Kaphanubandhi raktArsha	*Rakta Mokshana*
Pitta Vatanubandhi raktArsha	*Snehapana, Abhyanga and Anuvasana*
In Balavana Rogi	*Allowed to bleed to drain out Dushta Rakta*
In Durbala Rogi and Pittolbana RaktArsha in Greeshma ruthu	*Rakta Sthambhana*
After Shodhana of Dushta rakta	*Tikta Upachara for achieving Agni Sandeepana, Rakta Sangrahana and Dosha Pachana*

As the *Pitta* and *Rakta*, are in *Ashraya Ashrayee Sambandha*, the line of treatment of *Raktaja* also holds good for *Pittaja Arsha*.

Basti Chikitsa in RaktArsha – For *Raktasthambhanartha (Haemostasis purposes)* and to control the *Vata*, certain basti can be used as per the need like – *Pichha Basti*, *Ksheera basti*, *Prapoundarikadi Anuvasana Basti* etc.

Bahiparimarjana chikitsa in ardra Arsha

Lepa – When there is severe burning, bleeding from the protruded *Arshankura*, one should apply the *kalka (Paste)* of either

- *Manjishta / lajjalu + yastimadhu.*
- *Tila + yastimadhu*
- *Nimbarasa + goGhrita*
- *Madhu + Ghrita*

Parisheka **(Showering)** – To stop the excessive bleeding, *Parishechana of sheetajala* (Showering Cold Water) can be done after applying the *Guda Pradesha (Anal region)* with the mixture of *Sharkara* (Sugar) and *Goghrita* (Cow's Ghee).

Avagaha **(Sitz Bath)**– To alleviate the *Daha (Burning Sensation) and Kleda (Moisture)* to stop the *Raktasrava* (Bleeding), one can advise the *Avagaha* of either, *Yastimadhu sheetala kwatha (Cold Decoction of Yastimadhu), Sheetala Ikshurasa (Cold Sugarcane Juice), Vetasa Sheetala Kwatha or Sheetala Godugdha* (Cold Cow's Milk) after applying the *Sheetala Taila* (Cold Oil).

Aoushadhi Yoga in Arsha: Various drug combinations are mentioned in various classics, which should be used according to the *Dosha Pradhanata (Predominance of Humor involved in the disease pathology).*

Kshara karma (Chemical Cauterization by Plant Alkali): The procedures that utilise the *Kshara*, are mainly two, like *Pratisarana* (For external application in the form of paste) as well as *Kshara Sutra* (Medicated Barbour Thread, that is prepared by application of Alkali powder and other plant extracts), in case of the *Arsha*. The simple application of *Kshara*, over the *Mamsankura* for a stipulated period, will leave the *Dagdha* (burnt) area of the *Ankura* (Mass), which will fall off in succeeding days. Whereas, the transfixed *Kshara Sutra* around the *Arshankura*, induces the falling off of the *Ankura* by both the *Chedana (Excision effect) and Lekhana Karma (Scrapping Effect)*.

To facilitate, the procedure of application, the *Arshoyantra* (Proctoscope) is used both for the assessment of the growth of the *Arshankura*, as well as for the application of *Pratisarana Kshara* (Smearing of the paste of the Kshara or Alkali).

Arshoyantra (Proctoscopes and Colonoscopies):[38]

The yantra may be made up of metals, ivory or horns possessing the shape of *Gostana* (Nipple of Cow Udder), should be used to assess the disease as well as to do the procedures, like *Shastra (Surgical Excision), Kshara (Chemical Cauterization) and Agni (Thermal Cauterization)*. In males, the length is around four *Angula* (Length of Inter phalangeal joint of the Individual Self) and the diameter is of five *Angula* of each individual. In females, the length is equal to the length of her own palm and the diameter should be of six *Angula*. For the Diagnosis, the *Arshoyantra (Proctoscope)* with two openings measuring of three *Angula* length and width of one *Angushta* (Thumb) is used. Whereas, for the procedures, the *Arshoyantra (Proctoscope)*, with single opening is used. It is supported with *Karnika* (Demarked Side supports) Marks of half *Angula* projection, situated at the surgeon's end, about half *Angula* from the margin of the *Yantra* (Blunt Instruments).

But, the *Yantra* should be well selected, so that, it should be devoid of the defects (*Dosha*) like –selecting more wider or lengthier *Yantra*, when considering, the sex and built of that individual; or selecting the *Yantra* with small opening or with much wider opening, which will lead to misdiagnosis or improper procedure respectively. The surface of the *Yantra* should be smooth. Otherwise, a rough surface will cause *Marmaghata* (Injury to the vital part) and leads to pain.[39]

***Pratisaranakarma* (Smearing of Paste of Alkali)**[40]

The *Arshankura*, when passes the stage of *Bheshaja Chikitsa (Medical management)*, is subjected for the *Pratisarana Ksharakarma (Smearing of Paste of Alkali)*, irrespective of the predominant dosha, when it possesses the following features:

1. *Mrudu* (soft in consistency)
2. *Prasruta* (spread to the surrounding area)
3. *Avagadha* (deep seated)
4. *Uchrita* (projected)

Poorvakarma (Pre-operative Procedures):

- Patient should be nil by mouth on the day of procedure.
- Patient is supposed to take the food with *Snigdha, Ushna* and *Drava Guna Pradhana (More of Liquids)* properties and in little quantity, for the period of four to five days prior to the procedure.
- Patient is subjected to the procedure with all the routine operation theatre procedures.

Pradhanakarma (Operative Procedure):[41]

- The *Arshankura* is assessed with the help of *Dvichidrayukta Arshoyantra (Proctoscope)*, introduced into the *Guda Bhaga* (Anal Region) after the lubrication with *Ghrita* (Cow Ghee).
- Now *Ekachidrayukta Arshoyantra* (Slit proctoscope) is used. *Arshankura* projecting into the lumen of *Arshoyantra* is wiped with the sterile mop and *Mrudu Avagharshana* (Gentle Rub) is done, with *Shalaka (Probe), Gomaya Choorna* (Cow dung powder) or *Shefali Patra* according to the involvement of *Dosha*.
- The *Kshara* (Alkali paste) is applied over the *Arshankura* (Pile mass) of *Dakshina Bhaga* (right anterior) first. The thickness of the *Lepa* (Paste) is equal to the thickness of the *Nakha* (Nail) for *Pittaja Arsha*; twice the thickness of the *Nakha* for *Khapaja Arsha*. Whereas, three times thicker than the *Nakha*, is applied for the *Vataja Arsha*.
- The opening of the *Arshoyantra*, is closed and kept for hundred *Vakmatrakala*, (Time taken to count 1 to 100) to facilitate the burning process (Chemical Cauterization). Afterwards, the *Lepa (Application)* is wiped away, either with the *Dhanyamla*, *Dadhimastu (Curds supernatant)*, *Shukta* (Acetic Fermentation) or *Amlaphala Swarasa* (Juice of Citrus

Fruits), to assess the colour change in the Arshankura, as *Pakwa Jambu Phala (Colour of Ripened Jamun Fruit)* and *Kashmarya varna* in *Vataja Arsha; Mayura Kanta Varna (Colour of Neck of Peacock) in Pittaja Arsha* and *Brihati Pushpa Varna*, in case of *Khapaja Arsha*, which indicates the *Samyakdagdha lakshana* (Perfectly Cauterized)

- If the colour change has not occurred as expected, then the procedure is repeated till the expected colour change occurs.

Paschyatkarma (Post Operative Procedure):

- Apply burnt site with *Yastimadhu Ghrita* and advise the *Avagaha* of *Ushnodaka* (Hot Water Sitz Bath) in *Kapha / Vataja Arsha Rogi* and *Sheeta Avagaha* (Cold Water Sitz Bath) in *Raktaja / Pittaja Arsha Rogi.*

Precaution:

- One *Arshankura* should be treated at one time when there are multiple *Gudankuras*, that too in order of first of *Dakshina Bhaga* (right anterior), followed by the *Ankura* of *Vama Bhaga* (left lateral) and finally of *Prishta Bhaga* (right posterior), with a gap of one week duration in between each sitting.

Phalashruti (Result)

The *Vatanulomana (Regularization of Bowel Movement), Anneruchi (Tastefulness), Agnideepana (Improvement in Appetite), Bala (Improvement in Strength)* and *Varnotpatti* (Glow to Skin) and *Manasantushti* (Healthy feel) are indicative of properly done *Ksharakarma (Chemical Cauterization)*. Thus, the result obtained will be good.

Upadrava (Complications):

When the *Ankura (mass)* is burnt excessively, results into the *Upadrava* (complications) like *Daha (Burning Sensation), Murcha (Giddiness/Syncope), Jwara (Fever), Pipasa* (Excessive Thirst) and *Shonita Ati Pravrutti (Excessive bleeding/haemorrhage)*. Whereas *Heena Dagdha* (insufficient burn) may result into *Krishnashyama*

Varna {*(dhyama)*/ Bluish black colour}, improper burn, *Kandu (increased itching)*, *Vikruti in Anila (Flatulence and burping)* and disturbances in the *Indriya (Sensory organs)*.

Upachara (Management of Complications):

When the patient experiences *Shool* (Pain) in *Basti Pradesha (Hypogastric Area)* after *Ksharakarma*, should be treated with *Lepa* (Application) of the *Kalka* (Paste) prepared with *Punarnava, Kushta, Surabhi or Devadaru*. And if the patient experiences, Vibandha of Shakrut (Constipation) and Mutra (Urinary Retention), should be subjected for either *Parisheka* (Showering) or *Avagaha (Sitz Bath)* with the *Kwatha* (Decoction) of the *Varuna, Eranda, Gokanta* or *Punarnava* mixed with *Sneha*.

Kshara sutra (Medicated Surgical Thread of Alkali):[42]

The *Arshankura* with the features like

- *Chatrakara* (spread like an umbrella)
- *Urdhva visruta* (projected upwards from its base)

is subjected for the application of *Ksharasutra*, prepared by the repeated application of *Haridra Choorna* and *Snuhi Ksheera*. The *Kshara sutra* because of its *Chedana* (Excisional Property) and *Lekhana* (Scrapping Property) effect takes off the *Ankura*.

***Agnikarma* (Thermal Cauterization):**[43]

The application of the heat, to burn the Arshankura is decided on the basis of the following features:

- *Karkasha* (rough on touch)
- *Sthira* (firm at its base)
- *Pruthu* (fixed / not mobile)
- *Kathina* (hard in consistency)
- *Vata* or *Kapha Dosha* predominant

Poorvakarma (Pre-Operative Procedure):

1. Patient should be nil by mouth on the day of procedure
2. Patient is supposed to take the food with Snigdha, *Ushna* and *Drava Guna Pradhana* and in little quantity for the period of four to five days, prior to the procedure.
3. Patient is subjected to the procedure with all the routine operation theatre procedures.
4. Since, it requires the *Mamsa Dahana* (Cauterization of Muscle Tissue), the materials like either *Madhu (Honey)*, *Sneha (Oils and Fats)*, *Jamboshta* (Black Coloured stone type) or *Gud* (Jaggery) should be collected for the procedure.
5. The flame is produced by burning the coals of the *Khadira*, *Badara* etc. plants, by blowing with *Bhastrika (Blower)*. Then the *Jamboushta* is heated through this smokeless flame to red hot and is used for the application over the *Arshankura*.[44]

***Pradhanakarma* (Operative Procedure):**

1. Since the *Vataja* and *Khapaja Arsha* are to be burnt, which are *Sthira* (Firm), *Kathina* (Hard), *Pruthu* (Spreading) and *Karkasha* (Rough Surface), the type of burn used is *Pratisarana* (Smearing type) to take out the *Ankura* instantly from its root.
2. Since the *Arsha* is *Mamsapradoshaja Vikara (Disease of Muscle Tissue)*, the burn should be up to the extent of *Mamsa* (Muscle) and it should be done till it turns to *Samyakdagdha Lakshana* (Properly Burnt) like *Kapotha Varna (Pigeon Grey Colour)*, *Alpa Shwayatu (Less Post operative Oedema)*, *Alpa Vedana (Less post operative pain)* with *Shushka Sankuchita Vrina (Dry constricted wound)*.[45]

***Paschatkarma (Post operative procedure)*:**

Thus, the wound formed after the proper burning is applied with the *Madhu* (Honey) and *Sarpi* (Ghee)and left for healing.

Upadrava (Complications):

Upadrava due to the bad skills of the surgeon, one may end with the *Upadrava* like *Plushtadagdha* (insufficient burning), *Durdagdha* (improper burning) or *Atidagdha* (excessive burning).

Upachara (Management of Complications):

According to the condition, the measures that are mentioned in the *Agnikarma* context should be used.

Discussion on the relevance of Agnikarma in Arsha

Consideration of Vataja and Kaphaja Arsha for Agnikarma

Vataja and *Kaphaja Arsha* are indicated for the *Agnikarma* because of the opposite properties. The *Arsha* in the *Vyaktavasta* (Clinical Presentation) requires *Vyadhi Pratyanika Chikitsa* (Disease Specific Treatment) as *Chedana* (Excision) or *Lekhana* (Scrapping/ curettage). *Lekhana* can be achieved by *Pratisaraneeya Kshara* (Application of paste of herbal Alkali) but it takes more time. *Agnikarma*, superior to *Kshara* because of its action and as it doesn't allow the *Vyadhi* (Disease) to reoccur. It does the *Chedana* of the *Arsha*. The *Agni*, because of its *Ushna* (Hot) property subsides both *Kapha* and *Vata*. It also removes the *Ankura* (Mass), which is of *Mamsadhatu* / muscle tissue (*Prithvi Mahabhuta Pradhana*) from its root. Moreover, the pile mass consisting of venous plexus along with arterial twig from superior haemorrhoidal artery and certain amount of loose sub mucous and sub cutaneous areolar tissue surrounding the vessel, has got the tendency to bleed on excision. The *Agnikarma* ultimate one among the *Raktasthambana* (Hemostasis) measures, does both the *Chedana* of the *Ankura* and at the same time, *Raktasthambhana*. The External Piles, which bear the features as like the features indicated for the *Agnikarma* i.e, *Karkasha*, *Sthira*, *Pruthu* and *Kathina*, can be considered as *Vataja* and *Kaphaja Arsha*. Hence, they can be treated by *Agnikarma*.

Instrument and methodology:

Even though, the *Jamboshta Shalaka* (Probe prepared with the specific type of black stone) is mentioned for the *Mamsa* (Muscle Tissue) *Dahana* (Burn), the thermocautery with round tip also serves the purpose, as it is easily available and can provide well controlled heat as per the necessity. The Thermocautery probe is applied at the base of the mass to cut through smoothly by burning the tissue. This is like smearing off the base which serves the purpose of *Chedana* and *Raktasthambhana*.

A histopathological study of excised pile mass reveals as the specimen consisting of multiple dark brown tissue bits showing lining epidermis along with underlying loose areolar connective tissue with a few blood vessels and small bits of muscle fibers. The lateral and deep resected margins of the pile mass having the presence of necrotic tissue. Such a burn made deep up to the muscle fibers of corrugator cutis ani doesn't allow the *Arsha* to reoccur.

Effect of Agnikarma therapy on pain (*Ruja*)

Among the majority of the patients, pain will be most probably due to *Kaphavrita Vata* (Vata obstructed and covered by the Kapha) and in some patients, pain may be because of *Vidavrita Vata* (*Vata* obstructed by the stools or fecal matter). The relief from pain in such conditions can be achieved because of the local effect of *Agnikarma* in relieving the *Margavarodha* (Obstruction of the Vata for its regular movement) to *Apanavata* by the *Mamsankura Chedana* (excision of the Pile mass) and systemic effect of *Agni*, in liquifying the *Kapha* to take out the *Avarana* (obstruction or covering) to *Vata*. Thus, subsiding the aggravated *Vata* to relieve the pain. Administration of *Shatsakara Churna* and other similar laxatives and the purgatives, can help in relieving of pain, by relieving the increased intra rectal and intra anal pressure, that is by the impacted stools or the constipation (Relieving the *Vidavarana*).

Effect of *Agnikarma* therapy on *Kandu (Itching/ pruritus Ani)*:

As the *Kandu* (Pruritus Ani) is due to the *Karmatmaka Vikruti* (functional abnormality) of the *Kapha*, the *Agnikarma* helps by subsiding the *Kapha* because of its *Ushna* (Hot) and *Ruksha Guna (Dryness)*, that are opposite to *Sheeta* (Cold), *Snigdha* (Unctuousness) & *Kledata* (Moisture) of the *Kapha*. Further, *Kledayukta Kaphaja Arsha* are excised out to aid local effect of the therapy on *Kandu*.

Course of post – operative pain:

The post operative pain immediately after the procedure may increase but subsequently decrease after twenty-four hours. The increase in the pain immediately after procedure is due to the burning of tissue that results into necrosis. Patient's complaint of burning type of pain that may be attributed to *Rakta* and *Pitta Kopana* (slight change in the Blood PH and aggravation of the Pitta) by *Agni*. But application of medicated *Ghrita* (Ghee) relieves the pain (Daha / Burning pain) by the *Rakta Prasadana* (normalization of PH of the blood) and *Pitta Shamana* on 3rd day of post- operative period.

Course of *Vrina Srava* (raw wound discharge) after *Agnikarma*:

The *Vrina* (wound) has got minimal *Srava* (discharge) on procedure day which subsequently increases from 1st post operative day onwards as, the necrosed tissue gets separated from the healthy tissue in the form of liquified brownish black discharge. But the discharge reduces completely nil on 14th day. The absence of the discharge indicates the healed wound. The minimal *Srava* on the procedural day is because of the *Shushka Sankuchita Vrina* (dry constricted burnt wound) that is expected, as it is indicative of *Samyakdahana* (properly burnt wound). But, as the healing starts, the discharge increases on next day onwards for short period and gradually decreases from 3rd day onwards to complete cessation on 14th day as wound is healed.

Course of Vrina Varna (post Agnikarma raw wound colour):

The procedure, that results into dark coloured necrosed wound tissue turns to red pink with granulation on 3rd day. Wound colour which is pale pink on 7th day is almost completely replaced by skin colour by 14th day.

***Shastrakarma*:[46]**

The *Arshankura* bearing the features like

1. *Tanumoola* (thin base like a pedicle)
2. *Uchrita* (projected)
3. *Kledayukta* (discharging) are to be excised with the *Chedanakarma* or *Lekhanakarma*.

Poorvakarma (Pre operative Procedure):

- Is followed as of the *Ksharakarma* or *Agnikarma*.
- *Mandalagrapatra (Type of Surgical Instrument)* should be used for *Chedanakarma.*

Pradhanakarma (Operative Procedure):

The *Mamsankura*, which is big in size, occurring in *Balavanapurusha* (With Good Strength) is excised with *Mandalagrapatra*, followed by the *Dahana* (Burning/cauterization) with the red hot *Jamboshta yantra*.[49]

Paschatkarma: Similar to *Agnikarma*

Note: Improperly performed Shastra, Kshara and Agnikarma may result into Shandatva (Impotency), Shopha (Oedema), Daha (Burning Sensation), Mada (Delirium), Murcha (Syncope), Atopa (Flatulence), Anaha (Emptiness), Atisara (Diarrhoea), Pravahika (Dysentery) or even may result into Marana (Death). Hence one should be careful while applying the above measures.[48]

Pathyapathya (Compatible & Incompatible Regimen):

The *Ahara (Food)*, *Vihara* (Regimen) and *Pana* (Drinks), which help in *Vatanulomana (Regularizing the Bowel Movements)* and *Agnideepana (Improved Appetite)*, are to be used and opposite of these properties should be avoided.

Apathya (Incompatible):

The patient, suffering with or who has been cured of the *Arsha*, should avoid the following *Anna*, *Pana* and *Vihara* to avoid the trouble or the recurrence of the disease.

Table No. 11: *Apathya for Arsha rogi*

Ahara	***Vihara***	***Pana***
Shaka – masha, kareera, nishpava, bilwa, tumbi, pakvamra etc. *Mamsa - varaha, mahisha, mathsya, avi etc.* *Others – pinyaka, dadhi, pishtaka and food with guru and vishtambhi properties*	*Exposure to atapa, poorvi maruta, vamana, stri gamana,* *prishtayana, utkatakasana, vegavarodha and bastikarma etc.*	*Jala of prachya (western), avanti and aparantha rivers and guru jala.*

Table No. 12: *Pathya for Arsha rogi*

Ahara	*Vihara*	*Pana*
Shaka – patola, pattoora, rasona, grunjanaka, palandu, chitraka, punarnava, shoorana, tanduliyaka, ashwabala, vastuka, shunti, haritaki, bala, mulaka, asana etc. *Dhanya – yava, godhuma, raktashali, kulatta, shashtika shali, etc.* *Mamsa - Birds like shikhi, tittira, lava, daksha.* *For raktArsha – Shaka, - Palandu* *Dhanya – masura, mudga, adhaki, kushta, shashtikashali, raktashali.* *Ksheera, navaneeta, Ghrita and mamsa of aja (goat)* *Mamsa – aja, shashaha, harina, kapinjala* *For ShushkArsha – Shaka - trivruth,*	*Virechana, lepana, raktamokshana, kshara, agni & shastrakarma.* *Vatarsha - Snehana, swedana, vamana, virechana, asthapana, anuvasana.* *Pittarsha – Virechana* *Guda prakshalana – in shushkArsha is done by the sukhoshna kwatha of bhanga patra; sukhoshna jala.*	*Dhanyaka, nagara, panchamula, panchakola, ajaji, patha, bilwa siddha jala.* *Madira, sharkara, gouda, seedhu, takra, tushodhaka, arishta, mastu and shunti or kanthakari siddha jala.* *Vatarsha – hingwadi choorna siddha kwatha + pippalyadi Ghrita* *Pittarsha – prathak parnyadi siddha kwatha + Ghrita* *RaktArsha – manjishta, murungya siddha kwatha + Ghrita* *ShleshmArsha –*

danti, phalasha, changeri, upodika, shatavari, bakuchi, dadima dadhi siddha yamaka, nagara etc. *Mamsa – godha, lopaka, marjala, ashwavidh, ushtra, gomamsa, kurma etc.*		*surasadi kashaya siddha Ghrita*

Table No.13: *Summarized Chikitsa Upakrama of Arsha*

Kriya krama ***(Remedies)***	***Arsha bheda and avastha*** ***(Piles types & Stages)***
1. Bheshaja (Medicines) (a) *Bhallataka* is superior for (b) *Vatsaka twak* is superior for (c) *Kalasheya (Takra)* is superior for	*Alpa-dosha, lakshana, upadravayukta;* *Achirakalajata; Adrushya and drushya Arshankura;* *ShushkArsha (Vata and Kapha)* *ArdrArsha (Pitta and Rakta)* All types of Arsha
2. *Kshara (Alkali Treatment)* I. *Pratisarana (Smearing)* *(a) Teekshana pratisarana kshara* *(b) Mrudu pratisarana kshara*	*Mrudu, Prasruta, Avagada and Uchrita* *Vataja and Khapaja* *Pittaja and Raktaja* *Chatrakara and Urdhwa Visruta*

II *Kshara sutra*	
3. *Agnikarma (Thermal Cauterization)*	Karkasha, Sthira, Prathu and *Kathina;* *Vataja* and *Khapaja Arsha*
4. *Shastrakarma*	*Tanumoola, Uchrita and Kledavanti*
5. Raktamokshana	*Dushtarakta Sanchita Vata / Khapaja Arsha*

Fig. No. 16: Indication of therapy according to the *Ankura lakshana*

Mrudu, prasruta, avagada and uchrita
Indication - pratisarana ksharakarma

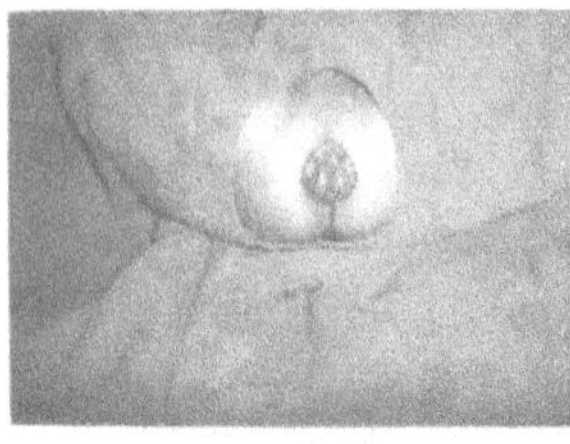

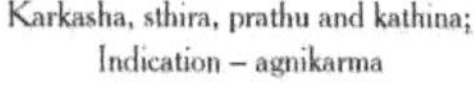

Karkasha, sthira, prathu and kathina;
Indication – agnikarma

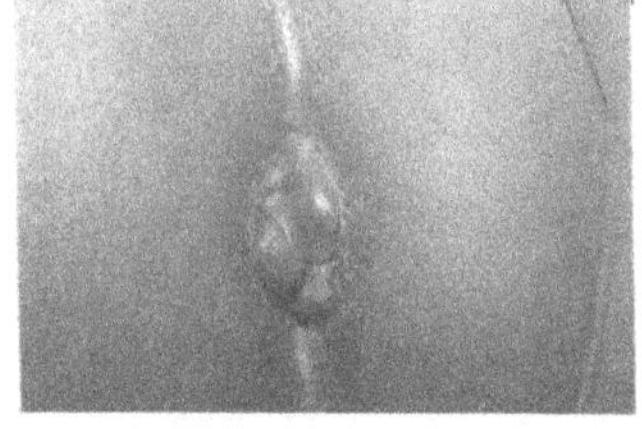

Alpa-dosha, lakshana, upadravayukta;
Indication – Bheshaja

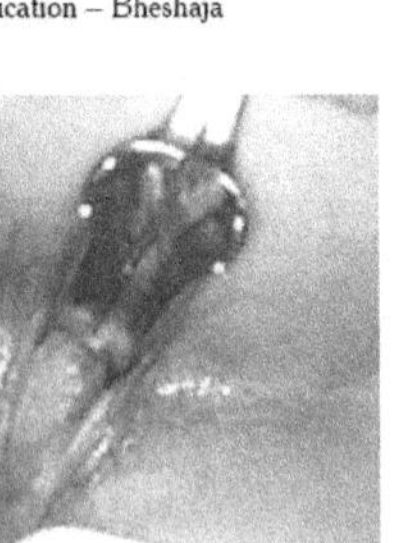

Tanumoola, uchrita and kledavanti
Indication – shastra karma

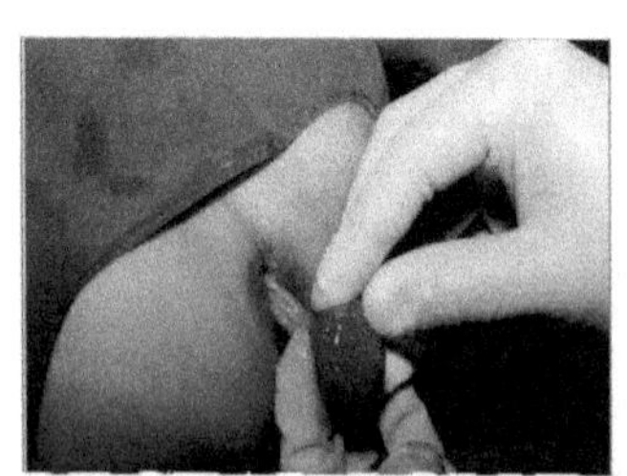

Dushtarakta sanchita Vata / Khapaja Arsha

Indication – rakta mokshana

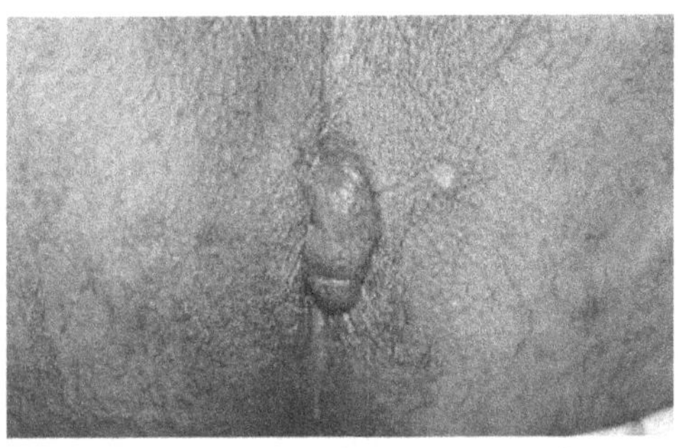

Summary

Most of the etiology that are mentioned in the context of the *Arsha* are of *Vata Prakopaka*, especially do the *Vilomagati* (moves the Vata to its opposite direction in the body and the channels) which is further assisted by the *Agnimandhya* (reduced appetite due to hypofunctions of the digestive system). So, the foods and drinks, which are *Ruksha* (dry), *Sheeta* (cold), *Guru* (heavy) and improperly cooked, aggravate the *Vata* by the their *Ruksha* and *Sheeta* property; aggravate the *Pitta* by their *Dravaguna* (liquid nature) and reducing its (Pitta) property of *Ushna* (hot) and its action *Pachana* (Digestive function); and the *Guru* (heavy) *Jalapana* (water that is heavy to digest), *Anupamamsa Sevana* (meat of cold climatic animals) etc, increase the *Kapha* thus, further diluting the action of *Pachakapitta* (digestive juices in the gut). The resulted *Ama* (undigested food and the resultant toxins) will interfere with the *Sara-Kitta Vibhajana* (separation of the nutrients and the wastes in the gut as well as at the subsequent levels of the metabolism). Thus, resulting into improperly formed *Pureesha* (Stools / fecal matter). Depending upon the predominance of the *Dosha*, the patient may experience *Baddha mala* / constipation and hard stools (because of *Vata*) or *Bhinna Varcha* / loose stools (because of *Dravaguna* /liquidity of Pitta).

The *Utkatkasana*, described as the position acquired by sitting such that, the *Parshnee* (heel) touching the *Prushtabhaga of Uru* (posterior of thigh), is nothing but the deep squatting position, that aids into the manifestation of the *Arsha* by increasing the intra-abdominal pressure.

Prishtayana (riding on the back of either animals or Bike riding) results into the pressure at the thigh region which obstructs the blood flow of venous return from the lower limbs. In addition to this the gravitational force is directly acting at the anal region because of which the blood is pooled in rectal veins to dilate them to produce the *Arsha*. Two-wheeler riding is the nearest comparison to this sort of *Nidana* and travelling for long distance also predisposes piles.

The vitiated *Apana Vata* in case of *Ama Garbhapata* (miscarriages / abortions), also vitiates the other *Dosha* to vitiate the *Mamsa Vali* (Anal mucosal folds) to produce the *Arsha*. The *Garbha Peeda* (pressure of gravid uterus on the rectum) can be considered as the definite organic obstruction to the iliac and superior haemorrhoidal veins.

The *Nidanarthakara Roga* (diseases leading to the Piles), like *Atisara* (diarrhoea) and *Grahani* (irritable bowel syndrome/ ulcerative colitis/ Crohn's disease/ straining at stools) associated with much tenesmus and futile straining may produce distending effect on the haemorrhoidal plexus to cause the *Arsha*. Moreover, the *Agnimandhya* due to *Atisara* and *Grahani* acts as the *Sannikrishta Nidana* (direct and effective cause) for the *Arsha*.

Pandu (chronic anaemia), when it is because of *Rasa Pradoshaja*, the *Shosha* (emaciation) occurs. Which, leads to *Mamsakshaya* (thinning and atrophy of the muscle tissue) because of which, the *Dhamani Shaitilyata* (tortuosity of vessels) takes place to cause *Mamsapradoshaja Arsha*. Whereas, the *Pandu* directly gives rise to *Shira Shaithilyata* (varicosity of veins) when it is because of the *Rakta Pradooshana* (vitiation of the blood).

The *Arsha*, since it is the resultant of *Agnimandhya*, the first and foremost *Dhatu* (tissue) involved is the *Rasa*, before the vitiated

Dosha could settle down in the *Mamsavali* at Guda (Anal mucosal folds). So, the *Poorvarupa* (prodromal features or pre-clinical stage) exhibited are of *Rasa Pradoshaja Lakshana*. But once the *Kamala* (Hepatobiliary diseases with Jaundice) or *Pleeha Vruddi (splenomegaly)* become the cause for the *Raktakshaya* (anaemia), then the *Vataja Arsha* manifest because of both *Dhatukshayajanya Vata Vruddi* (aggravation of *Vata* due to the tissue destruction) and the *Srotovaigunya* (defect in the channels of the body) i.e., *Sira Shaithilya* (varicosity of veins) due to *Rakta Kshaya*. And in *Roopa* (clinical features), the *Sarvangagata lakshana* (generalised features involving whole body) that occur are mainly because of the *Rasa Pradoshaja*. Thus, *Arsha* involves *Rasa (lymphatics)*, *Rakta (Blood)* and *Mamsa Dhatu (muscle)* in its manifestation with different systemic presentation.

So, paying due attention to the above-mentioned associated conditions of the *Arsha*, it can be considered that the *Arsha*, which is known as *Ari* (enemy) is definitely meant by the classics as secondary Haemorrhoids, in advanced conditions of the *Arshorogi (Piles patient)*. So, considering these *Arsha* with *Upadrva* (complications) as representing the different presentation of hepatic failure, one can understand the meaning or seriousness of considering the *Arsha* as one among the *Ashtamahagada* (one among the Eight fatal diseases).

Majority of the sufferers are male. This may be because of the more exposure to the *Nidana* of *Arsha* like bike riding, travelling, irregular food habit like *Vishamashana* (irregular and incompatible food habit), *Alpashana* (taking less quantity of food), *Anashana* (starving) and *Adhyashana* (excessive eating) and habits like smoking and alcohol which are *Pitta* and *Vata Prakopaka*, compared to females.

Majority of the non-vegetarian patients, may suffer with the Arsha Roga, who prefer the pork (*varaha*), chicken (*kukkuta*) and mutton (*avi*). These *Mamsa* are *Guru*, *Sheetala* and *Alpabhishyandhi* in nature to cause *Kapha Vriddi* and *Agnimandhya* to produce *Arsha*. More over the vegetarians who prefer more of Chana Dal, Toor Dal (Yellow Gram), Vathana

(Green peas), Potato, Wheat Roti, Ragi balls and shali do suffer from *Arsha because* of vitiation of *Vata* and *Koshtabaddata* (constipation).

Majority of the patients may notice pain at the anal region, either constant or related to defaecation, when the bowel is constipated. The *Kaphavruta Vata* (Vata obstructged or covered by the Kapha) that produces *Shaityata* (coldness/ dampness), *Gouravata* (Heaviness) and *Manda Ruja* (mild pain), may be attributed to the constant dull aching pain. Whereas, *Vidavruta Vata* (*Avarana* of *Vata* by the *Pureesha*) is responsible to produce the constipation and resultant pain as like *Parikartanavat* (cutting type of pain) at *Guda Bhaga* (Anal region).

Majority of the patients may have the complaint of *Kandu* (itching) at the *Guda Bhaga* of various grade, which not only indicates the presence of *Kandu* in only *Kaphaja Arsha* but also found in the *Vatakaphaja Arsha,* as the *Kandu* is due to *Karmatmaka Vikruti* of *Kapha Dosha*.

Note:

1. The *Nidana* that are mentioned for *Arsha*, remain same till today with little bit of modification like bike riding and distant travelling in place of *Prishtayana* etc.
2. *Arsha,* that occur associated with the *Udara* (Ascites / hepatic and splenomegaly), *Pandu* (Anaemia) and *Kamala* (Jaundice) etc, point towards the Haemorrhoids, secondary to the hepatic failure etc, systemic diseases.
3. *Bheshaja Chikitsa* (medicinal management), is useful in both the external as well as all degrees of Internal Piles. As a curative for the first degree and initial stage of second-degree Internal Piles and as a palliative treatment for advanced stage of the Internal Piles, for the patients, unfit for surgery or till the surgery is undertaken.
4. *Agnikarma* happens to be the ultimate treatment modality for the *Vataja* and *Kaphaja Arsha* (most often External Piles), that present with *Kathina (hard masses)*, *Parusha* (Dry

surface), Sthira (Stiff or firm) and Karkasha (Rough surfaced) *Lakshana* (signs).

5. *Ksharakarma* is indicated for the Internal Piles of First Three Degrees, presenting with the features of *Pittaja* and *Raktaja Arsha*, more predominant with the bleeding.
6. *Shastra Karma* (Surgical excision known as Haemorrhoidectomy), is indicated for both External Piles as well as Internal Piles of Second-, Third- and Fourth-degree Piles.
7. External Piles, most of the time, happen to be *Vataja* or *Kaphaja Arsha*. But, *Vataja* or *Kaphaja Arsha* cannot be only External Piles all the time.
8. Internal Piles, most of the time, happen to be *Pittaja* or *Raktaja Arsha*.
9. Never use cold water for cleaning the Anus, during the Fissure-In-Ano. Hot water wash is always beneficial for this condition.
10. Avoid Curds in all the case of the Anal Pathologies.

Part Two:
Review of literature on Piles / Haemorrhoids

9
Introduction

The haemorrhoids / piles are the one that interferes with the normal being of the persons with equal intensity, let it may occur as independent disease or as a sign / symptom of other diseases. This is a curse that has been donated to the human beings along with the gift that they adopted as erect posture.

The incidence itself indicates that it doesn't spare any age group and sex. Since the bleeding per rectum and the prolapse of the mass, disturbs the patient more than the pain, the aim of the treatment is directed towards dealing with the masses, thus indirectly dealing with the bleeding too.

But the complicated internal prolapsed piles, as the thrombosis and its sequel or more directed towards the conservative line of treatment according to the majority of the surgeons. Whereas the long standing prolapsed uncomplicated piles are dealt with surgical procedures-

Since the long time, many additions and modifications in the measures are being done to achieve the most beneficial effects with less hospital stay and post operative pain till today. But still the working surgeons are not satisfied. Even then, among the available treatment modalities, the formal haemorrhoidectomy happens to be the best one.

The chronic skin tags and external thrombosed piles even though are less severe, compared to internal prolapsed, but are given due importance as to reduce the pain, due to the clot in case of anal haematoma.

The recent addition like stappling method and laser surgery should provide the ray of hope to the hell of sufferers.

Since the present study is concerned to the external piles, the review of the internal haemorrhoids is delt in brief.

Incidence: The accurate idea about the incidence of the haemorrhoids is difficult. But the clinical observation suggests that very many people of both sexes suffer from haemorrhoids and that even more perhaps have piles in a symptomless form. But men seem to be affected roughly twice as frequently as women. The incidence of piles apparently increases with age and it seems likely that, at least 50% of people over the age of 50 have some degree of haemorrhoids formation. However, the disease is by no means confined to older individuals and are encountered in the people of all age, including the young children occasionally.

10

Anatomy[49] & Physiology of Anal Canal:

Anal canal commences at the level, where the rectum passes through the pelvic diaphragm and ends at the anal verge (the external or distal boundary of the anal canal) as it is the terminal part of the large intestine. It lies in the perineum in between the right and left ischiorectal fossae.

The anal canal is 3.8 CMS long. It is directed downwards and backwards. It is surrounded by sphincters which keep the lumen closed in the form of an anteroposterior slit.

The anorectal junction is marked by the forward convexity of the perineal flexure of rectum and lies 2 to 3 CMS in front of and slightly below the tip of the coccyx. Here the ampulla of the rectum suddenly narrows and pierces the pelvic diaphragm. In males it corresponds to the level of the apex of the prostate.

The anus, is the surface opening of the anal canal situated about 4 cm below and in front of the tip of the coccyx, in the cleft between the two buttocks. The surrounding skin is pigmented and thrown into radiating folds and contains a ring of large apocrine glands.

Relations:

Anteriorly the anal canal is related in the male to the apex of the prostate and to the membranous and bulbous parts of the urethra; in the female it is related to the lower third of the vagina. On each side the levator ani separates the anal canal from the ischiorectal fossa. Posteriorly the canal is related to the tip of the coccyx and to the anococcygeal raphae.

Muscles of anal canal:

The internal sphincter is a thickened continuation of the circular muscle coat of the rectum. This involuntary muscle commences where, the rectum passes through the pelvic diaphragm and ends at 6-8mm above the level of the anal orifice and 12-8mm below the level of the anal valves, where its lower border can be felt. The internal anal sphincter is 2.5cm long and 2-5 mm thick.

The external sphincter, formerly subdivided into deep, superficial and subcutaneous portions, is now considered to be one muscle. Some of its fibres are attached posteriorly to the coccyx, while anteriorly they are inserted into the mid perineal point in the male and in the female fuse with the sphincter vaginae. Unlike the pale internal sphincter muscle, which is involuntary, the red external sphincter is composed of voluntary (somatic) muscles.

The Longitudinal muscle is a continuation of the longitudinal muscle coat of the rectum intermingled with fibres from the puborectalis. Its fibres fan out through the lowest part of the external sphincter to be inserted into the true anal and perianal skin. The longitudinal muscle fibres that are attached to the epithelium, provide pathways for the spread of perianal infections and mark out tight compartments, that are responsible for the intense pressure and pain that accompany many localised perianal lesions. Beneath the anal skin, lie the scanty fibres of the corrugator cutis ani muscle.

*The inter sphincteric plane b*etween the internal (involuntary) sphincter and the external (voluntary) sphincter muscle mass, is found a potential space, the intersphincteric plane. It contains the basal parts of 8-12 apocrine glands.

The puborectalis maintains the angle between the anal canal and rectum and hence preserves the continence. There is a close association between the puborectalis portion of the levator ani and the external sphincter muscle.

The anorectal ring marks the junction between the rectum and the anal canal. It is formed by the joining of the puborectalis muscle, the deep external sphincter, conjoined longitudinal muscle and the highest part of the internal sphincter. The anorectal ring can be clearly felt digitally, especially on its posterior and lateral aspects. Division of the anorectal ring results into permanent incontinence of faeces. The position and length of the anal canal as well as the angle of the anorectal junction, depend to a major extent on the integrity and strength of the puborectalis muscle sling.

Interior of the anal canal shows many important features and can be divided into 3 parts like (A) the upper part, about 15m long (B) the middle part about 15 mm long (C) the lower part about 8mm long. Each part is lined by a characteristic epithelium and reacts differently to various diseases of this region.

Upper part (muscle membrane) is about 15mm long, lined by mucous membrane and is of endodermal origin. The mucous membrane shows 6 to 10 vertical folds; called as the anal columns of Morgagni. The lower ends of the anal column are united to each other by short transverse folds of mucous membrane called as anal valves. Above each valve, there is a depression in mucous called as anal sinus. The anal valves togaether form a transverse line that runs all around the anal canal. This is the pectinate line or dentate line.

Dentate Line is a most important land mark both morphologically and surgically. It represents the site of fusion of the proctodaeum and post allantoic gut and the position of the anal membrane, remnants of which may frequently be seen as anal papillae situated on the free margin of the anal valves. The dentate line separates

Above –Cubical epithelium	*Below* - From squamous epithelium
Autonomic nerves (insensitive)	From spinal nerves (very sensitive)
Portal venous system	From systemic venous system.

Middle part (Transitional zone of pecten) its length of 15mm is also lined by mucous membrane, but is devoid of the anal columns. The mucosa has a bluish appearance because of a dense venous plexus that lies between it and the muscle coat. The mucous is less mobile than in the upper part of the anal canal, refereed as pecten or transitional zone. The lower limit of the pecten often has a whitish appearance because of which, it is referred as the white line of Hilton. Even though, the white lie of Hilton is considered as easily recognizable, white and marks the interval between the external and internal anal sphincter, but there is absolutely nothing in the nature of a line white or of any other colour at this level and that can be recognised on inspection through a proctoscope or on examining an excised rectum.

The crypts of Morgagni are small pockets between inferior extremities of the columns of Morgagni. Into to several of these crypts, mostly those situated posteriorly, open one anal gland by a narrow duct. This duct bifurcates, and the branches pass outwards to enter the internal sphincter muscle in 60% of people. Issuing from this ampulla there are 3-6 tubular sub – branches that extend into the inter muscular connective tissue where they end blindly.

Lower part of Anal Canal: It is about 8 mm long and is lined by true skin containing sweat and sebaceous glands. The epithelium lining the upper 15mm of the canal is columnar (or stratified columnar) that lining the middle part (pecten) is stratified squamous, but it is distinguished from skin in that there are no sebaceous or sweat glands or hair, in relation to it. The epithelium of the lowest part resembles that of true skin in which sebaceous and sweat glands are present.

Arterial supply – Anal canal is supplied by branches from the superior, middle and inferior haemorrhoidal arteries. The most important is the superior haemorrhoidal artery, the terminal branch of the inferior mesenteric artery, whose left branch supplies the left half of the canal by a single terminal branch while its right has two terminal branches. The left and right middle haemorrhoidal arteries are the branches from the internal iliac arteries and right and left inferior haemorrhoidal arteries come from the internal pudendal branches of the internal iliac vessels. In general part of anal canal above the pectinate line is supplied by the superior rectal artery and the part below the pectinate line is supplied by the inferior rectal artery.

Venous drainage: - The internal rectal plexus (haemorrhoidal plexus) lies in the sub mucosa of the anal canal. It drains mainly into the superior rectal vein, but communicates freely with the external plexus and thus the middle and inferior rectal veins. The internal plexus is therefore an important site of communication between portal and systemic veins. The internal plexus is in the form of a series of dilated pouches connected by transverse branches around the canal.

Veins present in the three anal columns situated at 3, 7 and 11 o'clock positions (as seen in the lithotomy position) are large and constitute potential site for the formation of primary internal piles.

The external rectal venous plexus lies outside the muscular coat of the rectum and anal canal and communicates freely with the internal plexus. The lower part of the external plexus is drained by the inferior rectal vein into the pudendal vein. The middle part by the middle rectal vein into the internal iliac vein and the upper part by the superior rectal vein which continues as the inferior mesenteric vein.

Lymphatic drainage:

Lymph vessels from the part above the pectinate line, drain with those of the rectum into the internal iliac nodes. Vessels from the part below the pectinate line drain into the medial group of the superficial inguinal nodes.

Nerve supply:

Above the pectinate line the anal canal is supplied by the autonomic nerves both parasympathetic (pelvic splanchnic – S2, S3 and S4) and sympathetic (inferior hypo gastric plexus – L1 and L2). Pain sensations are carried by both of them.

Below the pectinate line is supplied by somatic nerves (inferior rectal S2, S3 and S4) thus convey the normal cutaneous sensation which is felt in the skin of the perianal region and of the wall of the anal canal below the level of the anal valves. This sensation can be abolished by an inferior haemorrhoidal nerve block.

Sphincter: The internal sphincter is caused to contract by sympathetic nerves and is relaxed by the para sympathetic nerves. The external sphincter is supplied by the inferior rectal nerve and by the perineal branch of the fourth sacral nerve.

Physiology of defaecation: Act of emptying the entire colon from splenic flexure through anal orifice is defaecation. This act is initiated by increasing the intra luminal pressure in rectum (20-25 mm water). The pressure receptor present in the rectum can differentiate the pressure due to gas, liquid or solid. The reflex centre is at hypothalamus, lower lumbar and upper sacral segment. Rectum is normally empty. The faecal matter is stored in sigmoid and pelvic colon, but not in rectum. The urge for defaecation develops as soon as faecal matter reaches rectum. In addition, the reflex of appropriate posture, voluntary relaxation of external sphincter and abdominal compression adds to the mechanism of defaecation. They are -

(1) Orthocolic reflex. - occurs when a person awakes from sleep assuming the erect position.

(2) Gastrocolic reflex. occurs when the person is moving and taking food and liquids. The increased intra rectal pressure causes the relaxation of anal sphincters, which is counteracted by voluntary contraction of external sphincter, permits the act to proceed. If the delay is prolonged, a temporary reduction in the intensity of the urge may occur.

VENOUS SUPPLY **BLOOD SUPPLY**

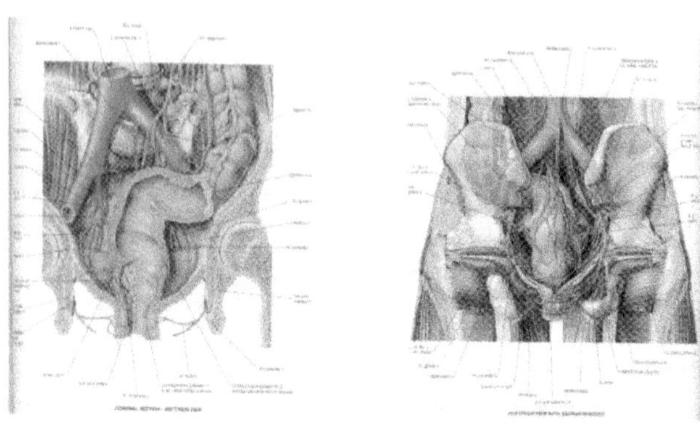

Fig: No. 17: ANATOMY OF ANAL CANAL

INTERIOR OF ANAL CANAL **MUSCULATURE OF ANAL CANAL**

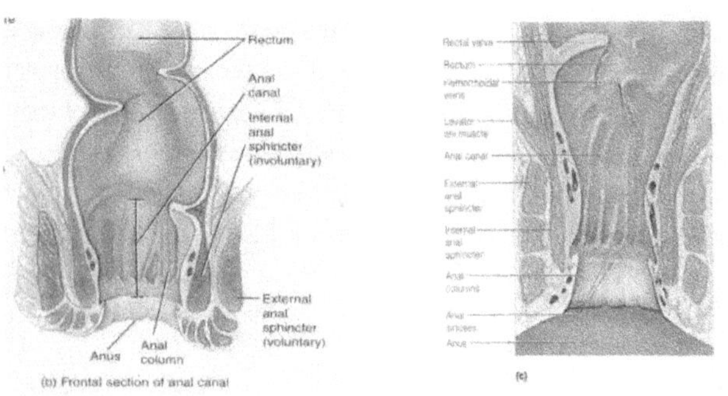

Fig. No. 18: Classification of Haemorrhoids

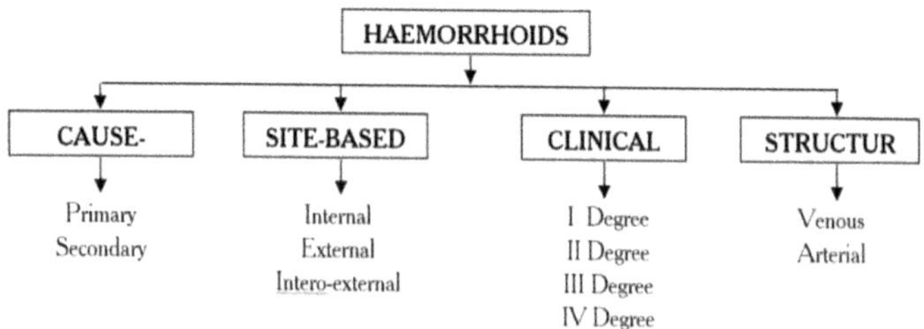

11
Etiological considerations

The aetiology of the internal haemorrhoids may be associated with a definite organic obstruction to the venous return from the superior haemorrhoidal veins or it may be idiopathic where, no evident organic venous obstruction is present.

The *definite organic obstruction* may be due to cirrhosis of liver; thrombosis of the portal vein and abdominal tumours, notably pregnancy.

Another mechanical cause of internal haemorrhoids frequently quoted is carcinoma of the rectum, as the presence of growth in the middle one third of the rectum obstructs the tributaries of the superior rectal veins in its wall and thus leads to venous engorgement and internal haemorrhoids.

Idiopathic:

Usually, it is impossible to ascribe the haemorrhoids to any particular cause, as the idiopathic cases represent the vast majority of patients. At the most that can be done is to point to a number of factors, which may have played a part in the production of the condition in any individual patient like

a. *Heredity*: The condition is so frequently seen in members of the same family that there must be a predisposing factor such as a congenital weakness of the vein walls or an abnormally large arterial supply to the rectal plexus.

b. *Anatomical* – Portal venous system is devoid of the valves so that in erect position the entire column of blood in the superior rectal, inferior mesenteric, splenic and portal veins from anal canal to liver bears directly on the internal haemorrhoidal venous plexus. Moreover, the collecting radicles of the superior haemorrhoidal vein lie unsupported in the very loose sub mucous connective tissue of the ano rectum. The superior rectal veins, being tributaries of the portal vein, have no valves.

c. *Physiological*: Compression of the superior haemorrhoidal veins during defaecation promotes the venous congestion as they lie in the sub mucous in the lower rectum or compressed by the descending mass of faeces, especially if the motion is hard and constipated. Further some degree of distension of the haemorrhoidal venous plexus in the anal canal is presumably an inevitable accompaniment of every act of defaecation. Hyperplasia of the corpus cavernosum rectum may result from failure of mechanism, controlling the arteriovenous shunts producing superior haemorrhoidal veins varicosity and haemorrhoids.

d. *Constipation, diarrhoea and straining at stool*: The distending effect of the normal defaecation on the haemorrhoidal plexus may be greatly magnified if the patient suffers from constipation as he has to engage in prolonged and repeated straining to pass large hard motions. Diarrhoea associated with much tenesmus and futile straining may also produce the same effect, but slightly less injurious.

e. *Diet*: The westernised food, which is devoid of the cereal fibres results into considerable delay in faecal transit time in the bowel and high incidence of chronic constipation.

f. *Deficiency of the anal sphincters / alteration of sphincter tone:* In patients who have had operations for anal fistulae involving division of a considerable part of the sphincters on one aspect of the anal canal, the venous plexus in the opposite wall, deprived of its normal support, frequently develops a haemorrhoidal swelling.

12
Pathogenesis

Internal haemorrhoids have been regarded as essentially varicosities of the venous plexus in the wall of the anal canal and lower most centimetres or so of the rectum. These bulge into the lumen of the anal canal, especially when the portal venous pressure is raised and the sphincters are relaxed during defaecation and straining.

The principal veins involved are those of sub mucous or internal haemorrhoidal plexus, which are mainly radicals of the superior rectal vein. In later period the subcutaneous / external haemorrhoidal venous plexus of the corresponding segment of the anal canal, also participate in the varicose process, resulting into an interno – external pile. Upper two third of such pile is above the level of anal valves covered with mucosa and lower one third lies below the valve covered with the skin of anal canal and anus.

Even though the dilated, tortuous veins are involved in the pathogenesis of the haemorrhoids, it is also associated with the sliding of the anal mucosa. The stretching or fragmentation of the muscularis sub mucosae ani results into the sliding down of part of the lining of the anal canal. Thus, it is clear that the any enlargement of venous plexus in advanced haemorrhoids might well be a secondary phenomenon consequent on sliding down of the mucosa.

In addition to veins, the contents of the pile include a small arterial twig (one of the ultimate branches of the superior rectal artery) and certain amount of loose sub mucous and sub cutaneous areolar tissue surrounding the vessels. Hence, the bleeding that occurs in connection with haemorrhoids is not dark and venous in nature but bright red. Internal haemorrhoids are frequently arranged in three groups at 3, 7 and 11 o'clock with patient in lithotomy position. This distribution has been ascribed to the venous drainage of the anus as veins present in the three anal columns situated at 3, 7 and 11 o'clock positions (as seen in the lithotomy position) are large and constitute potential site for the formation of primary internal piles.

Each principal haemorrhoids can be divided into three parts:

a. Pedicle: Situated at anorectal ring, covered with pale pink mucosa, occasionally a pulsating artery may be felt in this situation.

b. Body of the internal haemorrhoids commences just below the anorectal ring. It is bright red or purple and covered with mucous membrane. It is of variable size.

c. An external associated haemorrhoids lies between the dentate line and anal margin. It is covered by skin through which blue veins can be seen unless fibrosis has occurred. This can be seen in well-established cases.

An arterial pile may be produced as a result of haemangiomatous condition of terminal branches of superior haemorrhoidal artery entering each pedicle.

13
Clinical features

There are two cardinal symptoms of internal haemorrhoids like bleeding and prolapse. Pain is usually not a disturbing symptom unless, the pile is complicated with thrombosis. Discharge and anal irritation may develop in certain patients whereas secondary anaemia may get in due to excessive blood loss.

Bleeding: Bleeding is the principle and earliest symptom in first and initial stage of second-degree piles. In the beginning bleeding is slight streak on the motion, in the later stage, a steady drip of blood after defaecation. At still later stage, bleeding may occur apart from the defaecation at any time, when the piles prolapse and become congested.

Prolapse: is a later development. On the basis of prolapse the internal haemorrhoids can be classified into four stages as following.

1. *First degree prolapses* – In the earliest stage, the piles merely project slightly into the lumen of the anal canal when the veins are congested at defaecation.
2. *Second degree prolapse* - As time passes, the mucosal surface corresponding to the piles may appear externally, while the patient is straining but return spontaneously to the anal canal when the motion has been passed and the defaecating effort has ceased.
3. *Third degree prolapse* – At still later stage the piles prolapse even more readily and not only protrude during defaecation but remain prolapsed afterwards until they are replaced digitally within the anus.
4. *Fourth degree prolapse* – In long standing piles become so large and develop such considerable skin covered components that

they cannot be properly returned to the anal canal and remain as permanent projection of anal mucosa.

Discharge may be seen in the permanently prolapsed piles, associated with pruritis, which is most troublesome for the patient.

Anal irritation may supervene because of the moistening and soiling of the perianal skin from the discharge in the third-degree haemorrhoids. Even it may occur in other cases with less severe degree of prolapse.

Pain is absent unless complications supervene. Hence other associated condition should be suspected if any patient complains of pain.

The profuse bleeding from the haemorrhoids may cause the *anaemia*. The patient other than the features of piles presents with the breathlessness on exertion, dizziness on standing, lethargy and pallor due to increasing anaemia.

14
Examination

Is followed as routine for the rectal examination, along with the examination of the abdomen and if necessary, haematological investigations of any suspected anaemia.

Inspection:

First degree haemorrhoids do not usually produce any abnormality of the anal region that can be detected on simple inspection.

Mucosa of second-degree internal haemorrhoids is usually not projected unless the strain is exerted. But the skin covered components of the piles may be evident at the anal orifice as distinct swellings in the three main positions and most frequently on the right anterior aspect.

Large third-degree haemorrhoids will be recognised as projecting masses, the outer part of which is covered with skin, the inner portion covered with red or purplish anal mucosa. A linear furrow marks the junction, between the skin and mucosa. In long standing cases, as the mucosa stays in contact with cloths, the pannus, a white pale metaplasia of lining epithelium to a squamous epithelium, develops which extends from the mucocutaneous junction over the most dependent part of the mucosal surface and terminating in a rather irregular edge. In such advanced cases, the characteristic changes in the peri anal skin occurs that indicates pruritus ani.

Palpation:

In the early stages of the piles, as they are easily collapsible venous swellings cannot be perceived on digital palpation. But on long standing, as the sub mucous connective tissue undergoes fibrosis, the pile becomes palpable. It is felt as a soft longitudinal fold. Internal haemorrhoids also become palpable when they are thrombosed.

Gentle traction with the fingers on the loose folds of skin or skin covered swellings at the anal orifice often succeeds in drawing down some of the anal mucosa in case of second-degree haemorrhoids.

Proctoscopy:

It facilitates to assess the size and degree of the haemorrhoids. If haemorrhoids are present then they bulge into the end of the proctoscope like grapes when the patient bears down slightly and the instrument is gradually withdrawn. For this examination a proctoscope is passed to its fullest extent and the obturator is removed. The instrument is slowly withdrawn as the patient bears down, till the proctoscope just emerges from the anal orifice. At the end if there is no red anal mucosa is evident at the anal orifice then the piles are of first degree. But if the mucosa does project, then the piles are of second or third degree. The second-degree piles immediately slip back into anal canal out of the view and the anal orifice closes over them once the patient ceases straining. Whereas in case of third degree piles the mucosal prolapse persists after the cessation of straining till it is reduced digitally.

Sigmoidoscopy:

This becomes essential, when the proctoscopy reveals the absence of any significant haemorrhoids to account for the patient's bleeding, especially in patients of over 40 years of age to rule out the occasional presence of rectal or sigmoid carcinoma.

15
Complications of Internal Haemorrhoids

The two main complications of haemorrhoids are excessive bleeding and thrombosis with its sequels like fibrosis, sloughing, ulceration, abscess formation and rarely the portal pyaemia.

Strangulation is accompanied by considerable pain, which makes sitting on the part or having motion extremely uncomfortable. This state is known as "Acute attack of piles". Unless the internal haemorrhoids can be reduced within one or two hours, strangulation is followed by thrombosis.

Very rarely, after an attack of thrombosis the pile undergoes a dense *fibrosis* and projects as large fibroid mass at the anal orifice.

In certain cases, the thrombosis progresses to actual sloughing and *ulceration*. *Sepsis* may also occasionally occur apart from sloughing. Thus, formed abscess in the sub mucosa or in the perianal or ischiorectal region may be difficult to detect in the first instance.

16
Differential Diagnosis

A pile mass or haemorrhoids has to be differentiated from the following conditions

a. *Anal epithelioma:* A swelling characterised by pebble appearance, firm and nodular. Biopsy confirms the diagnosis.

b. *Condyloma accuminata:* This lesion is characterised by cauliflower appearance. Secretes more moisture with unpleasant odour.

c. *Condylomatum:* It is secondary lesion of syphilis. Warts like growth. Serological test is essential.

d. *Sentinel tag:* Generally situated in 6 o'clock position, always accompanies fissure in ano. It is so called because it stands guard.

e. *Hypertrophied anal papilla:* Firm masses arising from pedicle in dentate line.

f. *Pedunculated polyps:* Arise from mucosa of rectum and is painless.

g. *Sessile polyp:* These are true carcinoma. Biopsy confirms the diagnosis

h. *Haemangioma and Lymphosarcoma:* In both conditions' mucosa are coarsely pebbled but intact. Easily traumatised. Involvement does not confine to the zone of internal haemorrhoids.

i. *Rectal Prolapse:* Partial prolapse affects either a part or a circumference of anal outlet. The prolapsed portion is composed of longitudinal folds (centre to periphery) complete rectal prolapse is characterised by concentrically arranged mucosal folds.

Table No.17: showing summarized treatment modalities of piles

Method	Principle	Degree of Haemorrhoids
Diet modification	Soften stool, bulky stool by fibre; less straining	First
Sclerotherapy	Minor inflammation & fixation	First and second
Rubber band ligation	Moderate tissue destruction	First, Second and Minor Third
Infrared Photo coagulation	Minor tissue destruction and fixation	First and minor Second
Cryosurgery	Major tissue destruction and fixation	Second and third
Laser vaporization	Minor tissue destruction and fixation	First, Second and Minor Third
Laser excision	Minor tissue destruction and fixation	Third and fourth
Haemorrhoidectomy	Minor tissue destruction and fixation	Third and fourth
Dilatation of anus	Decrease the anal sphincter pressure	Second and third
Internal sphincterotomy	Decrease the anal sphincter pressure	Second and third

17
Treatment of Internal Haemorrhoids

Separate modalities are in practice depending upon the size and degree of haemorrhoids like -

- Expectant or medical treatment
- Injection treatment
- Rubber band ligation
- Manual anal dilatation
- Cryo surgery
- Infra-red coagulation
- Laser Surgery
- Stappling method
- Operative treatment – formal haemorrhoidectomy

Expectant or medical treatment:

The main aim of the medical treatment happens to be psychological aid to the patient as well as correction of other systemic symptoms due to the haemorrhoids, in small piles diagnosed in the routine examination of the rectum for the other complaints. Achieved by agents increasing bulk of stools, iron mixture, ointments and suppositories.

Injection treatment:

This measure causes the fixation of anal cushions to underlying tissue by means of injecting the sclerosing agents like phenol in olive oil or five percent phenol in almond oil etc. The sclerosing agent causes inflammation, fibrosis and scarring to fix the anal cushion. Helpful in first-degree internal haemorrhoids; small second-degree internal haemorrhoids; third degree internal haemorrhoids for the palliative purposes.

Rubber band ligation:

The rubber band ligated either with Barron rubber band ligater / McGivney ligater / Hoorn ligating proctoscope / Thomson's modified ligater causes the mechanical coagulation leading to sloughing off of the pile mass. Helpful in second degree internal haemorrhoids.

Contra indicated in first degree internal haemorrhoids and third degree large internal haemorrhoids with lower component covered with skin; ulcerative colitis, Crohn's disease and hypertrophied papillae.

Manual anal dilation (Lord's anal dilatation)

The internal piles are caused by circular constricting fibrous bands in the wall of the lower rectum or of anal canal. The forcible dilatation of anal canal and lower rectum helps to break these bands.

Cryo Surgery:

Necrosing the pile mass with extreme cold (up to –180 degree centigrade) applied with cryoprobe results into destruction of the mass.

Infra-red coagulation:

It is an elective treatment of piles for coagulating bleeding points by means of infra-red coagulator i.e., 14-volt wolfram halogen lamp with a gold-plated reflector.

Surgical treatment:

There are 5 varieties in formal surgical treatment - ligation and excision, submucosal haemorrhoidectomy, excision with suture, excision of the entire pile-bearing area with suture, excision with clamp and cautery.

The detailed technique of ligation and excision is -

Pre-Operative

1. Patient should be hospitalised 48 hours before operation.
2. Premedication as per requirement.
3. Soap water enema advised previous night and in the morning.
4. Diabetes mellitus and hypertension should be controlled well before the surgery.
5. Anaesthesia administered as required.

Operative

Patient is placed in lithotomy position with the buttocks projecting well beyond the end of the table and region is cleaned with antiseptic solutions. Sterile towel is spread over the region. Instrument table is arranged in convenient position.

Before proceeding with excision, manual anal dilatation to be performed gently. The pile is to be grasped with forceps, skin in relation to the primary pile mass is also grasped with another forceps and both the forceps are held together with one hand, with the help of pointed scissors, an inverted V-shaped skin cut is to be made. The subcutaneous tissue and sphincter are separated by gauze dissection. Then the root of the pile mass is ligated well and excised. Then the trans fixation of the stump is to be performed. The final appearance of operated area should resemble the three-leaf clove. The wound should be absolutely dry before applying dressing. Then cotton wool is applied and 'T' Bandage is tied.

Post Operative

Dressing is to be left undisturbed for 24 hours. Afterwards it should be changed twice daily. Final healing takes several weeks, liquid paraffin is given daily evening; to minimise the pain, analgesics may be employed.

Complications could be reactionary haemorrhage, skin tag formation, stenosis and anal stricture, retention of urine, abscesses, fissure in ano, incontinence of faeces, prolapse of lower rectum.

18
External piles and Its Management

These form at or just outside the anal orifice. The mass is covered with skin, endowed with ordinary cutaneous sensation, thus troubles the patient with extreme pain and their complications.

Classification:

1. Acute thrombosed external piles or anal hematoma
2. Chronic anal skin tags.

Chronic anal skin tags are classified into idiopathic and secondary.

Thrombosed external piles:

Thrombosis of blood in the veins of the external subcutaneous haemorrhoidal plexus renders the name, thrombosed external pile.

Pathology:

It is assumed to be a rupture of one of the external veins during straining at defaecation with escape of blood into the subcutaneous tissues. Where it clots and forms a dense painful swelling giving the name anal hematoma.

But histological examination of an excised anal hematoma confirms the clot with an endothelial covering supporting the postulation of the formation of hematoma not extra venously.

Signs and symptoms:

- Sudden development of a painful lump at the anus aggravates by defaecation and sitting.
- May be accompanied with bleeding due to rupture of the hematoma.
- Swelling is covered with the tense stretched skin through which bluish colour of the contained clot is visible.
- In early stages swelling is more tender which diminishes after a week.
- Multiple hematomas may occupy the greater part of the anal circumference.

Sequel –

- Spontaneous resolution may occur resulting into reduction in the pain and swelling.
- Rupture of haematoma may occur followed by complete extrusion of the clot.
- Exposed clot may get infected to form fistula or abscess.

Treatment –

Expectant Treatment:

- Majority of anal hematoma soon become painless and usually absorbed without incident. Thus, the following measures assist for the same
  - Bed rest
  - Sitz bath (hot)
  - Sedatives
  - Laxatives

Operative treatment

- Evacuation of the clot either under short general anaesthesia or local analgesia with very short incision i.e., radially placed.
- Clot is squeezed out between the finger and thumb.
- Post operative care includes frequent sitz baths and dry cotton wool pad over the anal region for a few days.

Anal skin tags:

These are exceedingly common around the anal orifice, may be single or multiple may vary from a slight excrescence of skin to grossly projecting tags.

Classification – *Idiopathic* skin tags

- Secondary skin tags

Idiopathic skin tags:

- These are not associated with any obvious causal condition.
- May or may not possibly represent a legacy of resolved haematoma.

Clinical Features – Soft and pliable and are covered by normal skin.

Treatment - No treatment is required except in large skin tags, which cause nuisance to the patient in cleaning the anal region after defaecation or discomfort.

- Under LA excision of the tags is done to leave a flat pear shaped or triangular open wound which cannot fail to heal satisfactorily by granulation.
- Associated internal piles including skin tags as much as possible are excised by the formal haemorrhoidectomy.

Secondary skin tags – Usually secondary to anal fissure or pruritus ani.

Clinical features – Skin tags associated with fissure in ano are normally stiff with oedema when the fissure is open, which becomes flaccid after healing of fissure.

- Skin tags associated with pruritus ani will be oedematous and presents with infected skin rugae and the anal and perianal skin changes.

Treatment – Is directed to the causal factor either fissure or pruritus ani.

<u>Differential Diagnosis:</u> - Anal warts

- Condylomas
- Carcinoma

Part Three:
From My Clinical Experiences

19
How to Identify It?

The Pain, Bleeding and the feeling of Abnormal Growths or Swellings at their Anus, make the persons apprehensive and force them to visit their doctor, coming out of their shyness or initial hesitancy. They become more fearful, as their ass is not visible to them and they are not sure, what exactly burning their ass. Some of my patients were smart enough, that they clicked a selfie of their Anus and rushed to me, horrified by the look of the new swellings at their most important part. More than the ingestion, normal excretion, keeps our body healthier. And it is undisputed that, all the excretions give you immense pleasure, especially, when they were withheld for the longer time.

Now days, because of the advancement in the technology, most learned patients, Google about their problems, before coming to the doctors. This practice is creating much more problem, rather than the relief. Medical Science cannot be as straight as the simple mathematics. Here 2+2, cannot be 4 always. It can be 1,2,3,5 or anything. Because, the same complaints may be secondary to many of the different pathological conditions. But unfortunately, persons get themselves mislead by the artificial intelligence and the mind is so subtle and quick to respond to all such situations that, it may recreate exactly the same Signs and Symptoms, that are read over by the patient, even though, the real pathology may be different in him. This impact on their subconscious mind will not allow the medicine to act to their fullest potency and that further worsens the condition. The patient goes into the vitious cycle of the misconceptions in the mind- to the presentations of the same symptoms that he misunderstood- leading to no relief from the complaints- creating more fear and belief in the misconceptions- thus, more aggravated Signs and Symptoms. Hence, to be honest with you, many a times I felt that, medical information on the internet need to be more precise and a disclaimer should be popping up on the screen and a suggestion for the reader to contact their doctor, before scrolling down to the information.

Ayurveda believes that, a disease can be diagnosed only when, the main three examinations are done. They are 1. *Darshan Pareeksha* (Inspection of the patient by the doctor), 2. *Sparshan Pareeksha* (Touch/ Palpation of the patient by the Doctor) and 3. *Prashna Pareeksha* (Interrogation / Questioning the patient regarding their complaints).

Ironically, the one which is the third and last step of the examination, The *Prashna Pareeksha* (Examination by Interrogation) is being used first by the patients themselves, that too to an Artificial Intelligence, and the Final Diagnosis is arrived by the patient himself, most of the time, the wrong one, complicating the situation.

So, any pain in the Anus, cannot be always with Haemorrhoids, rather the **Haemorrhoids, most of the times are painless, unless they are complicated with either inflammation or thrombosis. Bleeding even though the hallmark of the Haemorrhoids**, but it can also be seen in the conditions of **Fissure-in-Ano, Rectal Polyp** and even in the **Carcinoma of Sigmoid Colon, Rectum and the Anus**. **Prolapse of the mass from the Anal opening can be Haemorrhoids, Rectal Polyp or even the Rectum itself. Discharge** from the anal canal can be the mucous, pus, pyo- sanguineous (pus mixed with blood) and mucous- sanguineous (mucous mixed with the blood) because of Hypertrophied Anal Papillae, Peri Anal and Ischio-Rectal Abscesses, Fistula-in-Ano, Ulcerative colitis, Crohn's Disease respectively.

So, the *Arsha* (Piles / Haemorrhoids) with the cardinal features of 1. Abnormal Growth, 2. Discharge, 3. Bleeding and 4. Pain, can be any of the diagnosis as mentioned above, which satisfy all the four cardinal features of the Arsha. But, **the nearest diagnosis for the *Arsha* is taken as the Haemorrhoids or Piles, the**

Rectal Polyp and the Anal Condyloma / Anal Warts. The Carcinomatous growths are dealt under the heading of the *Arbuda* (Tumour), by most of the Ayurvedic Surgeons. Rectal prolapse is named as *Guda Brimsha* in Ayurveda. The Fissure- In-Ano is called as *Parikartika* and the Peri Anal and Perineal Abscess are contexed under the *Vidradi.*

Differential Diagnosis: Usually, the Haemorrhoids can be easily identified by their appearance, but only when they become evident. But, by then, the Haemorrhoids would be in the advanced stage, requiring the Surgery. The Piles are classified into Three types as 1. External Piles, 2. Internal Piles and 3. Interno- External Piles.

The External Piles are outside the Anal canal and Anal Verge, covered by the skin and are non-Bleeding. They are usually painless, unless complicated with the Thrombosis, secondary to the rupture of the smaller branches of external subcutaneous haemorrhoidal plexus followed by the extravasation of the blood space below the skin and forming the clot. The patient will present with the tender, painful and firm swelling outside the Anal verge, with Bluish Red or Brick red in colour.

The Internal Piles are called as Piles, when they are non-Bleeding and called as the Haemorrhoids, if they are Bleeding. The Internal Piles, that are covered with the Mucosal covering, are categorised into 4 Stages called as First- Degree, Second- Degree, Third- Degree and the Fourth- Degree. Some Authors and Surgeons merge the Third and Fourth Degree and have only Three stages of the Piles.

The First-Degree Piles are the one, which are the initial stage of Piles, confined to the Anus. They are not visible outside the Anal Canal, but can be made out by the Proctoscopic Examination by the attending Surgeon. These Piles are the resultant of the sliding of the Anal Mucosa and are more prone for Bleeding, if contain much prominent varicose veins in it. At this stage, the patient feels mild discomfort in the Anus and Heavyness in the Rectum and dropwise bleeding while defection.

The Second -Degree Piles are the one, that come out of the Anal Canal while defecation and return back to the canal once the stools pass off the Anal verge. Patient feels this movement of the Pile mass. In the initial stage of the Second Degree, the bleeding is more prominent with the streamwise pattern.

The Third -Degree Piles, come out of the Anal Verge, but fail to return back to the Anal Canal. Patient replaces this mass manually. Interestingly, the bleeding tendency reduces drastically due to the fibrosis of the mucosal covering of the Pile mass. Whereas, **The Fourth -Degree Piles** are prolapsed outside and cannot be replaced inside the Anal Canal and may lead to the complication of the Thrombosis and are then called as the Prolapsed Thrombosed Piles. Bluish Red colour of the mucosa suggests of the presence of the blood clot beneath the mucosal covering. The later stage of Second Degree to Fourth -Degree Piles undoubtedly require Surgery. **So, don't get misled by the commercial advertisements of some Ayurvedic Pharmaceuticals, claiming the cure of the Piles without Surgery.** So, the intelligence is to identify the disease in its preclinical stage, so that the Surgery and its consequences can be avoided.

If, the patient repeatedly complains of either of any of these problems, related to their Gut, like Bowel Gurgling, Flatulence in abdomen, Anorexia, Constipation, Sour belching, burning sensation in the Abdomen, Excessive burping, Irritable Bowel Syndrome, Crohn's & Ulcerative colitis, should be careful and be observant towards their Bowel Habit. If they notice any associated complaints like Heavyness, Itching and Cutting type of Pain in the Anal region, should be looking into the colour, consistency and odour of the faeces. Improper bowel evacuation along with hard stools may increase the chance of getting the Haemorrhoid. Also, the semisolid or watery stools with increased frequency per day, has got equal incidence of causing Haemorrhoids. If the person is already suffering with the Anaemia, Hypoproteinaemia, Chronic Cough, Ascites, Benign Prostatic Hyperplasia, any obstructive conditions of Urine-Flatus-Stools, Bronchial Asthma and other

Chronic Obstructive Pulmonary Disorders and Chronic Insomnia and if his bowel habit gets altered, then have got more chance of getting into the pathology of the Piles.

Bleeding:

The first and foremost Sign of the Haemorrhoids is the Bleeding Per Anus. But the Bleeding is also seen in the conditions like Fissure-In-Ano, Rectal Polyp, Rectal Prolapse and the Carcinoma of the Rectum. But it may not be the same in case of Piles.

But, looking into the pattern of the Bleeding, one can easily differentiate the Haemorrhoids from rest of the above-mentioned conditions of the Bleeding. In Haemorrhoids, the bleeding will be either dropwise or streamwise. In the First Degree and initial stage of Second Degree, the bleeding is mostly dropwise and in the late stage of the Second Degree and the initial stage of the Third-Degree Haemorrhoids bleed in stream.

If, the streak of blood on the stools is seen along with the burning pain at the Anal region, it will be **Fissure -In-Ano**. Dropwise as well as stream like bleeding is also present in the **Rectal Polyp**, but it is mostly found in the paediatric age group. It looks like a lollypop, red in colour and gets spontaneously into the rectum after the defecation. It is freely movable in the rectum and Anal canal on digital examination by the Surgeon, due to its long pedicle.

Carcinomatous Anal Tumour, will be more prone for bleeding, either dropwise or ooze on touch. **Rectal Carcinoma** will bleed like splash on pan, at the onset of the defecation. Patient feels the urge for the defecation, once the Rectum is stretched by the collection of the blood overnight, along with the stools and passes the dark red blood as of splash on the pan of the toilet. **Rectal Prolapse** also ooze out the blood, but not a prominent complaint.

Appearance:

The Haemorrhoids/ Internal Piles will be usually, either pink, when they are non-bleeding and in their initial stage; red when they are congested and inflamed; pale white when they are covered with the fibrosed mucosa or bluish black and mixed with the red colour, when they are prolapsed and thrombosed.

Rectal Polyp will be like red lollypop. **Rectal Prolapse**, is pink and sometimes red when congested, and is a circumferential prolapse. Whereas, the prolapsed Piles will be segmented in appearance, as they are placed apart in their primary and secondary positions.

The Fissure-In-Ano with the sentinel pile is presented with a linear ulcer at the anal verge and a skin appendage at the base of that ulcer. It usually occurs in the 12 o'clock and 6 o'clock position of the Anus, if it is compared to a clock, where in, the 12 o'clock lies towards the anterior part of the Anus towards the genitalia and the 6 o'clock is the posterior side of the Anus towards the tail bone.

The external piles are covered with the skin, firm and are placed in the primary and/ or secondary positions of the Anus (Primary positions represent the 11 o'clock, 3 o'clock and 7 o'clock of the imaginary clock at the Anus, with the assumed position of the patient in the lithotomy position. Whereas, the secondary positions are 1 o'clock, 5 o'clock and 9 o'clock at the imaginary clock of the Anus). **They never bleed,** but present with a dark red or bluish black coloured mass, when they are thrombosed. Anal warts and Condyloma also appear like the external Piles but will be of irregular shape, spreading and with rough surface, not restricted to the primary or secondary positions of the Piles.

The Anal carcinomatous growth will be hard to touch, ferocious appearance by its colour and bleeds on touch. **The perianal abscess** will be just adjacent to the anal verge, swelling appears associated with the fever and throbbing pain will be there. Again, the position may not be fixed to the primary or secondary positions of the Piles. These can be differentiated from the External

Piles as the abscess has got sudden onset of diffuse swelling with the preceding fever and throbbing pain. The colour change of the surface is not much evident compared to the Thrombosed external piles, which are bluish red or blackish red in colour with a definite demarcated boundary of the swelling. **The Fistula- In- Ano,** will be presented with an opening on the surface of the perineum, discharging the pus. **The Hypertrophied Anal Papillae** are the tiny teeth (Canine tooth) like white structures inside the anal verge, increasing the mucous discharge and causing the severe itching at and around the Anus, due to the irritation of the skin by the mucous.

Pain:

The pain in and around the Anal region, is experienced by the patients in multiple conditions related to the Ano- Rectal and Buttock area. Usually, the Piles are painless unless they are complicated as mentioned earlier. The First-Degree and Second-Degree piles, will not have pain except some discomfort and heaviness in the Anal region. The discomfort and heaviness are secondary to the increased Intra Anal Pressure and the congestion at the Pile mass. The Third- Degree and The Fourth- Degree internal piles, lead to intolerable pian due to their prolapse and the strangulation by the Anal sphincters and the Anal Verge. The External Piles will give acute severe pain, overnight, due to the Thrombosis, otherwise, they are painless. The Sentinel pile is usually painless, unless it is inflamed.

If the patient complains of severe burning pain after the defecation, then it will be often due to the Acute and Chronic Fissure-In-Ano. Whereas, Throbbing Pain is indicative of the peri-Anal and Perineal Abscesses. The Fistulous boil, before the formation of the fistula and the closed Fistula opening with the collection of the pus in the Fistula Track, may also cause the throbbing pain, but with mild intensity, compared to the Abscesses. Moreover, the history of the repeated incidence of pain followed by the pus discharge will be confirming the Fistula- In-Ano.

Anal warts and Condyloma of Anal region will be more prominent with the Pruritus Ani (Itching at the Anal region) rather than the pain. Proctitis (Inflammation of the Rectum and Anal canal), will be annoying the patient with the burning pain and discomfort, whole day. The malignant growth of the Anal Canal and Rectum are painless in the initial stage, but gives discomfort and pain, once they get local infiltration of the surrounding structures.

Summary:

So, on simple and keen inspection, we can make out, Perianal and Perineal Abscess by the colour change of the over lying skin into red or brawny red colour. The Thrombosed External Piles, by its bluish black tinge on the Skin Surface of the Pile mass and are differentiated from the Thrombosed Prolapsed Internal Pile Mass, by the same Bluish Black tinge over the Mucous Membrane Surface. The Fissure-In-Ano, can be seen as a linear (Line like) Ulcer (Wound), more commonly at the midline or in line of the median raphe. The Fissure is placed in the Anal verge and can be seen by giving a small stretch at the Anal Verge. Many a time, the Fissure can be associated with a small skin appendage, **the Sentinel Pile,** which will be with skin wrinkles/ creases, that may obliterate, when, the Sentinel Pile is inflamed and swollen. Fistula-In-Ano can be made out by the presence of a small hole that represents, the opening of the Fistula Tract.

If, patient feels pain on touch to the part, then it is called as Tenderness, as it gives pain on touch. The tenderness is always secondary to the inflammation. The Thrombosed Piles (Both Internal and External), the Abscesses, Pus filled Inflammed Fistula Track and the Inflammed Sentinel Piles will be painful on touch.

Soiling of the undergarments and discharges are usually because of the ruptured Perianal/Perineal Abscesses; the discharging Fistula and Sinuses and Increased mucous secretion due to the Hypertrophied Anal Papillae.

The Part One and Part Two of this book might have given you clear idea regarding the Piles of different type and stages, if you have gone through those sections. If, you have not gone through those sections, then I suggest you to go through those sections to have better understanding about the Piles and you can see the images to identify them easily.

20
How To Prevent It?

When, the man could evolve from his nearest and assumed ancestors, like the **Human- Chimpanzee,** and acquired more erect posture, started walking on the Two limbs (Bipedalism), the nature, even though blessed the humans with the many of the gifts, at the same time, probably cursed him with the Haemorrhoids. So, because of our built as well as our lifestyle, we are more prone for this disease. The anatomical reason of the lack of the valves in the portal vein, and effect of the specific gravity of the Earth on the Rectal, Mesenteric and Portal veins, are considered as the basic reason for the incidence of the Haemorrhoids/ Piles in us compared to the quadrupeds.

As, already there is more vulnerability is towards having the Haemorrhoids, the factors that hamper the normal drainage of the venous return of the blood from the Anal region, will double the chance of manifestation of the disease. The weak musculature of the Anal wall and mucosa along with the walls of the veins, get worsen by the causes, that put more strain on these musculatures. So, we need to avoid all those ill habits that aggravate the muscle weakness, varicosity of the veins and should adopt the good habits, that maintain the normal tone and strength of all these muscles.

Healthy habits of Food and other our daily physical activities, provide the good strength to the muscles of the Gut and help the endocrine and exocrine glands to function normally. Thus, avoiding or delaying the manifestation of the Haemorrhoids. The Hereditary cause along with the other acquired causes, can also be overcome by adopting the healthy habits as prescribed by the Ayurveda in the form of *Dinacharya* (Daily regimen) and *Rutucharya* (Seasonal regimen) with the prescribed diet and physical activities.

Physical Activities:

"The more you sit, the more you will lose the chance of sitting comfortably in your life in future."

The sedentary life style, will help and accelerate the basic mechanism of manifestation of the Haemorrhoids. The prolonged sitting and standing at one place will increase the retrograde pressure of the Portal Vein on the Rectal Veins, because of the slow or impaired movement of the venous blood column towards the heart. The locomotion of the limbs has got their influence to stimulate the gut movement and these gut movement have their further impact on the movement of the blood vessels in the form of their contraction and relaxation. This mechanism is not happening when we do not move. Further, the effect of specific gravity, worsens the condition to lead to the pathology of the Haemorrhoids, both functionally and structurally. So, to keep yourself free from Haemorrhoids, you need to have the minimum ten thousand steps of walking per day and changing your position at least Half an Hourly or Hourly, when it is inevitable to avoid the prolonged sitting position, because of your profession and other conditions. **Take a Hundred Steps after your Food, at least a must after the dinner.**

The *Sarvangasana* (*Yogasana* Posture with your Legs, buttocks and lower back upwards in straight line, perpendicular to the earth plane, supported by your shoulders, scapular region and head resting on the ground), practiced starting from Two minutes, gradually increasing up to maximum to Forty-Five minutes every day, on empty stomach, once you are back from your whole day's sitting or standing work, will protect you from getting the Piles. Sleeping on your left lateral side after food will reduce the incidence of the Haemorrhoids, by proper digestion of the food.

Heavy weight lifting (more than your capacity) without the abdominal supporters; Straining at the defecation, especially on the western latrine pot (commode); and working with your upper limbs, that requires extra pressure and strength, while sitting in the deep squatting position for longer period, all these acts, increase the intra

-abdominal pressure. The increased intra- abdominal pressure will increase the retrograde pressure on the Rectal Veins, leading to the anal mucosal sliding down along with the varicosity of the rectal veins. Try to be grounded in the *Sukhasana* (sitting on the ground with your Anus, both outer side of the ankle bones and lateral sides of the lower legs touching the floor, legs crossing each other, folded at the knee and hip joints) as much as possible, especially while taking food and doing some household works. This position, not only avoids the incidence of Piles, but also improves your appetite, functions of all the glands (Both Exocrine & Endocrine), normalizes hormonal functions and you will never suffer with the Hyper-acidity and gastritis, which is one of the causes of the Piles.

Defecation:

The defecation is to be kept normal as much as possible. Normal defecation is always of two physiological mechanisms, 1. Orth- Colic Reflex, we get the urge for the defecation, when we get up from our bed in the morning. The bowels, sense the change in the position of the body from lying to sitting up. This movement stimulates the peristaltic movements of the intestines and that creates the urge of defecation, second one is 2. Gastro-Colic Reflex, is generated on first intake of a glass of water, a cup of tea or after the breakfast. Even, some of have developed the habit of having this reflex on smoking or chewing Tobacco or Gutkha (tobaccos variant in India). Again, here the onset of the peristaltic movements, is induced by the movement of the first part of the Gastro-intestinal part that is the Mouth and the Oesophagus. When, either of these two mechanisms are working for you, then it is well and good. But, if you try to do either of the two following forceful acts, with respect to your defecation, then, you will yourself, invite the Haemorrhoids in your life. **So, avoid 1. Supressing the natural urge of the defecation and 2. Inducing forceful defecation.**

1. **Supressing the natural urge of the defecation-** misleads our body physiological functions, the bowels get confused by your act of the suppression of the urge. The intestines are programmed to throw out the metabolic wastes before, the

waste becomes injurious to the internal environment of it. The *Apana Vata* (responsible for the excretion of the Faeces, Urine, Flatus and Semen) is moving in its normal course of clockwise and downward direction, following the course of the Large Colon, to execute the defecation. But, by withholding this act, you are obstructing the normal movement of the *Vata*, then the turbulence is created in the Anal canal first, which further moves upwards, that is in the opposite direction of the expected normal course of movement of the *Apana Vata*. This increases the, intra- Anal, Intra-Rectal and Intra-Colonic pressure, compressing the veins lying in the walls of these parts of the colon, leading to the impairment of the venous drainage and increase in the retrograde pressure on the most dependent veins of the Colon, that is the Rectal veins and their tributaries, causing the varicosity in them, which will be prolapsing out, alongside the Rectal and Anal Mucous, which is already sliding down due to, either weaker musculature or by excessive straining at the defecation, as in the second case, as below (Inducing Forceful Defecation).

2. **Inducing forceful defecation**- this act is against the normal function of the body. Many a times, for our own convenience, before leaving our home for the professional duties, we try to attend the lavatory, even though there is no nature's call for the defecation. In normal conditions, as long as there is no required amount of the distention of the Rectal walls, the urge for defecation will not arise. But, as I said, for our belief that we should finish off the defecation, before taking the bath or before leaving for a long journey or a professional meeting, we try to forcefully induce the act of defecation, which forces the aggravated action of the *Apana Vata*. This aggravated *Apana Vata*, exerts the pressure over the musculatures of the whole Colon, Rectum, Anal and the walls of the vessels, that are supplying and draining form these structures through the *Vyana Vata*. This unexpected and undue pressure, causes the sliding of the Anal mucosa, allowing the tortuous rectal veins to herniate into the mucosal slide, that present as the Haemorrhoids or the Piles.

The frequent and long-term habit of either Suppressing or Forceful inducing of the natural urges of the Faeces, Flatus and Urine, will have important role in causing the haemorrhoids and also the diseases of all the system. So, neither suppress the natural urge of defecation nor forcefully induce it, if you want to be free from the Haemorrhoids. **As much as possible, try to attend the defecation urge in the deep squatting position rather than the chair position, over the commode. The deep squatting position has the advantage over the position on the commode, as it gives easy pass away for the stools by straitening colonic curvatures and adds supportive muscular pressure from the abdominal wall over the colon and rectum to do their act of defecation easily. Also, it prevents the occurrence of Inguinal Hernia, that may be the resultant of over straining at the defecation, in the persons with weaker musculature of abdominal wall.**

Sleep:

Sound and timely sleep, will keep the body younger and healthier. Altered and deficit sleep invites early aging and other health issues due to the reduced immune power. Scientifically, eight hours of sleep per day is considered as ideal, to keep yourself younger and healthier. Even, if you take eight hours sleep, but not at the right time, then, that also is one of the major causes of many diseases.

"The Late-Night Sleeps and Day Time Sleeps", both are injurious to health.

The regular habit of going to bed and sleep at late hours of night, aggravate both the *Vata* and *Pitta.* The aggravated *Vata* dries up the bowel and hardens the stools/ faecal matter. The aggravated *Pitta,* causes the gastritis and duodenitis, even subclinical inflammation of the Gastro-intestinal Tract, leading to the weakness of the gut wall musculature and altered functions of the bowel. Weaker Gut wall musculature is further strained by the forceful straining to pass the hard stools down the colon. This strain of the muscular wall leads to the sliding of the Anal Mucosa and Varicosity of the rectal veins. Thus, causing the Piles.

Even the Day time Sleep, that too immediately after taking the food, will cause the same pathological consequences, as mentioned above due to the aggravation of the *Pitta*. The Day time sleep is not indicated for every individual. It is only for the children, pregnant lady, old aged, ill health people and for the people that work in the night time. Even, the people working in the night can take the day time sleep on empty stomach, that too for the period of half of the night sleep, that they are deprived off.

So, even the normal individuals and the patients of Haemorrhoids, Fissure-In-Ano and Fistula-In-Ano, should "**Avoid the Late-Night and Day Time Sleeps.**"

Sex:

Sex is the integral part of every individual. But, excessive indulgence in the Sex may increase the chances of manifestation of the Piles/ Haemorrhoids. The excessive sex aggravates both the *Vata and Pitta Dosha* and leads to the same pathophysiology for the formation of the Haemorrhoids as discussed in the above/ earlier section of the Sleep.

The Sex during the period of sufferings with the haemorrhoids, increases the complaints of Burning and Bleeding per Anus. The Ayurveda classics suggest that, one shouldn't indulge in the sexual act, till he is free from the Piles. The complete sexual abstinence is indicated for the period of one year, even in the Fistula-In-Ano. The Patient experience, the sudden increase in the burning pain of the Fissure-In-Ano, immediately after the Sex. So, avoid the Sex, when you are having the episodes of acute events of the Piles, if you want to control and cure your Haemorrhoids at the earliest without the intervention of the surgery.

Seasonal Exposure:

"Too much is always Too Dangerous." The prolonged and excessive exposure to extreme Hot Sun will cause the *Pitta Prakopa* (aggravated *Pitta*), that causes the subclinical inflammation and dehydration of the cells of the gut. Thus, leading to weakness of the gut wall. This leads to increased permeability of the blood vessels and thus, leading to the bleeding per Anus. The excessive exposure to extremely cold climate, aggravates the *Vata Dosha* by the cold property. This reduces the rate of normal digestion in the gut, resulting into the improper digestion of the food. Thus, stools are not properly formed and it becomes too hard due to the dry property of the aggravated *Vata Dosha*. The mobility of the bowel is also affected, compelling of straining at defecation and thus pushing the weaker and lax mucosa of the Anal canal, down as Piles. Always we should follow the Seasonal Regime as mentioned in Ayurveda, to keep ourself disease free. Look into the Part One of this book for the details of the regime, that to be avoided in particular season, to avoid the Haemorrhoids.

Avoid excessive exposure to extreme cold and hot climate to prevent yourself from the Piles and Haemorrhoids respectively.

Habits:

Habits in excess are always the definitive as well as accelerating aetiologies for the Haemorrhoids. The excessive intake of Tea, Coffee, Alcohol, Tobacco, Gutkha and excessive smoking all contribute equally for the production of the Piles.

Drinking Tea on the empty stomach as well as frequently, causes its long-term bad effect over the Mucosa and Musculature of the Alimentary canal. Its astringent taste, called as the *Kashaya Rasa* in Sanskrit, has got the *Sthambhana* (Stoppage or restriction of the movements in the body, with respect to the tubular structures and the liquids in the body channels) property, which reduces the bowel movements and by that promotes the hard stools. The more time the stools remain in the large colon, the more fluid absorption from that in the colon occurs, causing hard stools. Hard stools are the reason for the excessive straining by the patient at the defecation and it is the cause for the mucosal injury in the Anal Canal, causing bleeding from the haemorrhoids and Fissure-In-Ano.

Alcohol also has the *Kashaya rasa* and moreover, the alcohol is known for its influence to facilitate the hampered functions of the liver, Intestines and the pancreas. The improper digestion of the food and the portal vein hypertension, secondary to the Alcoholic Liver Cirrhosis, lead to the formation of the Piles and even the secondary Piles. The liver pathology, further leads to the altered clotting factors functions, increasing the bleeding tendency of the haemorrhoids.

The Coffee, Tobacco, Cigarette and Gutkha, all are *Katu in Rasa* (Pungent in taste) and Hot in potency. They aggravate the *Pitta* and further course of the formation of the Haemorrhoids follows, as discussed above in the context of Sleep and Seasonal exposure.

Avoid Excessive intake of Tea, Coffee, Alcohol, Tobacco, Gutkha and Cigarette to Avoid Chronic Anaemia and Haemorrhoids.

Food and Drinks:

The basic principle behind selecting or avoiding a particular food or drinks is very simple. Your food should not aggravate either the *Vata, Pitta* or both of them. The *Kapha* is less potent in producing the Haemorrhoids, so the food stuff aggravating the *Kapha,* may not immediately produce the Piles. Moreover, the *Kapha Prakopaka* (*Kapha* Aggravating) foods are less taken in our food because of their tastes like Sweets, Salty and Sour stuffs.

The Indian Continental foods are much rich in fibres and scientifically designed with much verity to suit all the seasons and constitutions. But sticking to same food throughout the year, without changing, as per the season, produce the Haemorrhoids.

Most of us are fond of some food stuffs, that we include that in every slot of our daily intake. That food or drink may not be suitable to certain seasons, as they may accelerate the aggravation of the particular *Dosha,* which is already in its natural course of the aggravation due to that particular Seasonal effect. Foods and their seasonal selection will be the vast topic to deal. So, we cannot explain all here. But, **out my clinical observation, I have enlisted the following foods and drinks that are to be either limited or completely stopped when you are suffering with Haemorrhoids.**

1. Potatoes- as it aggravates the *Vata Dosha.*
2. Brinjal – It aggravates both the *Vata and Pitta.*
3. Cereals – like fresh peas ***(Pisum sativum),*** *Chana dal* (split yellow gram / desi chickpeas), The Indian *Toor Dal* (split pigeon peas) or the Yellow Gram (*Cajanus cajan*), the cow pea (*Vigna unguiculata*) or black-eye pea.
4. Fruits: most of the foods can be taken, except the **bananas** and **the sapota or chikoo**. The bananas and the Chico have got the property to get fermented, once they come in contact with the gastric juices. That is what is called as the *Abhishyandhi* (Fermented). But usually, the patients start taking the excessive of the Bananas, once he notices some pain in the Anal region and troubled with the constipation. This increases the Burning pain and Bleeding tendency of the Haemorrhoids. **So, avoid excessive intake of bananas, when you are suffering with the constipation associated with the bleeding and Pain per Anus.**
5. Curds do have the Abhishyandhi property that worsens the burning pain and bleeding per Anus in the presence of either Haemorrhoids or the Fissure-in-Ano.
6. Chicken, Pork and the Mutton
7. Green chilli and Tomato.

Take Moong Dal (Green Gram), Ghee, Milk, Butter, Buttermilk, Rice, Jawar, maze and plenty of All leafy vegetables. As much possible, the wheat bread should be avoided during the problem. If, it is unavoidable, then, the wheat bread be taken with the vegetables with more curry. All the fruits and vegetables can be taken, except that have been mentioned to be avoided as above.

21

How to cure it?

The stage of the disease will decide the management. The initial stage of Second- degree and the first- degree Piles / Haemorrhoids, can be best managed by the Ayurvedic Medicines. Whereas, the Third-degree and Fourth -degree Piles / Haemorrhoids are the definite indication for the Surgery. However, Ayurveda gives unique measures in the form of para-surgical procedures named as *Kshara Karma (Chemical Cauterization), Kshara Sutra (Alkali applied Thread) and the Agnikarma (Thermal Cautery)*, that can deal with the Piles of all the first Three-Degrees. The Surgical intervention is a must for the fourth- degree piles as per Ayurveda too. **(For the details of the medicines and the other treatment procedures kindly refer Chikitsa chapter in Part One and Treatment Chapter in Part Two, for Ayurvedic and Allopathic measures for the Piles, respectively).**

First-Degree Piles: This can be prevented from leading into the next advanced stages as well as can be cured, by following the regimen of food, sleep and physical activities that are mentioned earlier, in the chapter of **'How to Prevent it?'** Hot water sitz bath, after defecation as well as at least twice a day, will be soothing the pain and discomfort of the Piles as well as the other conditions, like Fissure and Fistula in Ano. The constipation and the flatulence should be relieved by using the medications as per the constitution of the person and the type of the gut.

For, the Piles patient of **Vata predominant constitution with the Hard stools and without bleeding,** one can use the following drugs from the Ayurveda- 1. *Dashamoola Kashaya* (decoction of the group of Ten herbal drugs) 20-30 ml twice in a day with 30 ml of Luke warm water, on empty stomach, preferably, morning 7 AM and evening 7 PM, 2. *Erandamooladi Kashaya*, 3. *Abhayaristha*, 4. *Ashwagandharistha*, 5. *Draksharistha*, 6. *Pippalyaddhyasava* etc., any of them as per the prescription, can be taken in the same dosage and timing as same as of *Dashamoola kashaya*, 7. *Triphala Guggulu*, 8. *Nimbadi guggulu*, 9. *Arshogna Vati*, *10. Sooranadi vati*, *11. Kravyadi Vati*, any of one of them, Two tablets each time, twice a day again preferably at morning 7 AM and Evening 7 PM, on empty stomach.

The granular preparations like *Manibadra Guda*, *Haridra Khanda*, *Eranda Bhristha Haritaki*, *Lavanabhaskara Choorna*, *Trivrut Choorna* and *Kalyanaka Ksahara* and many of the patent Ayurvedic laxative powder preparations for Piles and Haemorrhoids (except kshara) can be usually taken, One to Two spoonful before Dinner with Luke warm water.

For, the patients with the Pitta predominant constitution, having the loose stools with the Bleeding Piles/ Haemorrhoids, should be administered with the Ayurvedic preparations like, *Kutajaristha* or *Mustakutajaristha*, 20 to 30 ml with equal water of room temperature, twice a day before food. The *Bilva Avaleha*, *Kushmanda Avaleha*, *Manibhadra Lehya*, *Kutaja Phanita*, *Kanakayana Vati*, *Rasa Parpati*, *Bahusala Guda*, *Sukumara Gulika*, *Kankayana Vati*, *Avipattikara Choorna*, *Navayasa Choorna*, *Ushirasava*, *Panchavalkala Kashaya*, *Panchatiktaka Ghrita*, *Panchatiktaka Guggulu Ghrita*, *Shatavari Ghrita*. The dose and the timings vary person to person, hence should consult the Ayurvedic surgeon for the same.

The only precaution to administer the *Asava* and *Aristha* preparations is that, the patient should not be having Heartburn or Sour belching.

Second Degree Piles/ Haemorrhoids: initial medical management is same as of the first-degree Piles. The *Vatanulomaka* (Laxatives / Carminative), *Sukha Virechaka* (Purgatives), *Agnideepaka*, *Balya*, *Shotha Hara* drugs are administered, in the non -bleeding Piles associated with the Hard Stools or Constipation. Whereas, *Sangrahi*, *Agnideepaka*, *Pitta Shamaka*,

Rakta Prasadaka drugs are to be given in the Bleeding Piles or Haemorrhoids associated with the loose stools.

If, the masses are prolapsing out, then best option is to get rid of it physically. Ayurveda offers, best remedies like Kshara Sutra Ligation (Thread ligation medicated with the herbal Alkali and other herbal materials and latex) of the mass and Kshara Pratisarana Karma (application of herbal alkali paste) to shed off the masses, by mechanical cutting and chemical cauterization, respectively. Also, contemporary science offers, Infra-red coagulation, Laser treatment, Cryosurgery, Rubber band ligation and Haemorrhoidectomy.

Third- and Fourth-Degree Piles: The Third- Degree Piles finds it's indication for the *Kshara Sutra and Kshara Karma*. The Haemorrhoidectomy is the treatment of choice in much bigger masses covered with the Fibrosed mucosa, in Third-Degree Piles and Prolapsed Thrombosed Piles of the Fourth- Degree. The pain alleviation and reduction in the inflammation of the Prolapsed Thrombosed Piles, can be achieved by application of Ice cubes wrapped in a gauze piece, over the prolapsed masses, as a first Aid, before surgery. Even hot sitz bath, in certain cases gives the temporary relief.

External Thrombosed Pile Mass:

If, the mass is small and less dense, with less severe pain, then oral medications can be tried like *Kanchanara Guggulu, Kaishore Guggulu* along with potent Analgesic and Anti-inflammatory drugs from the contemporary science. But, if, the mass is bigger in size with much dense consistency and blackish discoloration of the over lying skin, then surgical excision of the thrombus (clotted Blood), is inevitable. Throughout the course, the Hot Water Sitz Bath is very effective.

Fissure-in-Ano, is the most common Anal condition, that needs a mention here, as it is most often thought, as if it is a Piles by the laymen. The fissure is totally different from the Piles. It is a linear Ulcer at the Anal verge. Mostly, season dependent and recurring condition, causes severe burning pain at the Anal region, often patient get confused and feared it as the Piles.

Most of the time, it does not require any surgical intervention, unless it is so severe to cause fainting / syncope to the patient, during defecation due to its pain. Otherwise, simple Ayurvedic medicines, that help the softening of the stools and healing of the ulcer, should take care of the patient. **Best and half the treatment is the Hot water Sitz Bath**, after each defecation or minimum three times a day, even with the normal bowel frequency. **Avoiding the Curds, Tea, Coffee, Alcohol, Tobacco, Spicy Food, Bananas, Yellow Gram, Potatoes, Day time sleep, late night sleeps and Sex, are found to be more effective in relieving the pain.**

The concept and usage of *Matra Basti* (Administration of the Luke warm, medicated Oil or Ghee with a catheter and syringe at the amount of 30 to 60 ml per day through the Anus, after the food) with either the *Yastimadhu Taila, Ksheerabala Taila, Prapoundarikadi Ghrita and other Madhura Ghana Sidda Taila and Ghrita* can be used for instant relief of the pain. Even simple application of the *Goghrita* (Cow Ghee) or *Shatadhouta ghrita,* is most effective in the fissure, even in the infants and the children.

The external applications on the external Piles are ineffective, as per my observation. Whereas, they may have much help in the Internal piles with respect to reducing the bleeding and soothing in case of the inflamed and congested haemorrhoids. But, if anybody claims, that mere application of any ointment will make the Piles to shed off, then that should be critically evaluated, before accepting the application.

22
Epilogue

The right awareness at the right time, can create wonders for the life. Little bit of care towards our own body and mind will definitely keep us free from the diseases and gifts a healthy and long life. The health is a real wealth as it paves the path, for the success in our life. **Ayurveda is the real-life science with its Two main objectives 1. Preservation of health of a healthy individual and 2. Curing the diseased.**

If, we follow the instructions and the daily and seasonal regimen prescribed by the Ayurveda, we can prevent ourself from the acquired diseases, like the Haemorrhoids. As, every individual is more prone to acquire the Piles, that is usually precipitated by the wrong life style and food habits, we need to adopt the regimen of the Ayurveda as per the day and the season.

The best options are available for all the diseases, when they are detected in their earlier stage. The unique list of the earlier symptoms, related to the Gut, as prescribe in the Ayurveda, helps us to keep a track on our bodily changes and thus, we can prevent the diseases, especially the Haemorrhoids. So, the repeated symptoms, like loss of appetite, hyper acidity, flatulence, constipation, loose stools, sour belching, excessive burping, all of these are the initial indication of the onset of the pathology at the Gut and the reflection of that pathology, as a Pile or Haemorrhoid at the Anal region. The best way to prevent yourself from the Piles is to decide your food and daily activity, based on your Gut feeling. Your Gut, gives you the indication for its needs and don'ts. Try to follow the instructions that are laid down in this book in the context of "**How to Prevent it**" and for more detailed understanding, about the Ayurvedic principles about the pathology and its treatment, kindly refer the Part One of this Book.

If, your job requires prolonged sitting, easy manoeuvre of contracting and relaxing your Anal Sphincter, at least Ten times a day with the focus at the anal region, even while you are working, will reduce the chances of getting afflicted by the haemorrhoids, significantly.

If you notice any discomfort like the heaviness, itching, cutting type of pain or burning at the anal region, don't hesitate or postpone to visit your doctor. If, the right diagnosis and the right medication is done at this early stage, will definitely prevent you from developing the Piles, provided life style and food modifications are made as per Ayurveda. So, feel free to discuss with your doctor, regarding these lifestyle modifications. Many a times, most of the doctors, only give a prescription of a laxative, analgesic and at the most an antibiotic (this type of practice is more prevalent in India), without giving much emphasis on the real causes, that origin from the food and the life style errors. Thus, advancing you to the next degree of Piles and its consequences of complications and demand for the invasive procedures. If, you find your doctor is not concerned about enquiring and correcting your food habit and the faulty life style, then, better change the doctor, especially to a Shalya Specialist, the Ayurvedic surgeon.

"Unless, you avoid the Aetiologies, you cannot avoid the Disease". So, be vigilant about your aetiologies by going through the Part One and the Part Three of this book and try to avoid them, even if, your attending doctor fails to evaluate them.

If, you are late to diagnose your Piles, then as per the stage or degree of the disease, you can opt for the treatment options available in Ayurveda, before going for the Haemorrhoidectomy, unless it is inevitable. For, more clear indication and opting for the treatment modalities, you can once again visit the Part One and the section of "How to Cure it" from the Part Three of this book.

Be aware and vigilant about the probable complications and their consequences, before trying medicines on your own, without taking a confirmed diagnosis from a well experienced surgeon. **The wrongly understood Perineal Abscesses, as an external**

Piles, can lead to the Fistula; mis diagnosed growths at the anal region as Piles may turn out to be an Anal Carcinoma. Even though, this book has made its best efforts to educate you to understand the Haemorrhoids and Piles, both by the Ayurvedic and Allopathic Perspective, but an expert opinion always makes the difference, especially when that opinion is combined with the tips of this book.

Even though, Part One of this book may feel disengaging and a difficult read for the non-Ayurvedic persons, still I request you to read it thoroughly, as the treasure of Ayurvedic remedies, not only for the Haemorrhoids, but also for all other life style disorders are hidden in it.

Of course, Ayurveda has got more options of less invasive measures and cost-effective medicines to treat the Piles, without giving a room for the recurrence of the disease, if judiciously applied.

I have made my best efforts to make Ayurveda and its remedies to be easier to understand by providing that extra chapter of "**Some Basics of Ayurveda for the Beginners**". So, go through that chapter repeatedly if you get confusion or stuck during your read of this book. The main goal of this book is to prevent every individual from acquiring Piles and thus to change the algorithm of its prevalence.

Hope this reading has added an extra inch of value to your knowledge, to help yourself and the others.

Bibliographic References

1. J. Goligher JC ; Surgery of Anus Rectum and Colon ; Baillire Tindal, London, 5 edtn; PP 98
2. Vagbhata; Ashtangahridaya; with commentaries of Sarvangasundara of Arunadatta & Ayurveda rasayana of Hemadri; annoted by Dr. Anna Moreshwar Kunte & Krishna Ramachandra Shastri Narve; edited by Pt. Hari Sadashiva Shastri Paradhakar; Chaukhamba Surabharati Prakashana; reprint 2002; Nidana Sthana 7/2; pp 490
3. Sushruta; Sushruta Samhita; with Nibandha Sangraha commentary of Sri Dalhanacharya, edited by Yadavji Trikumji Acharya; Chaukhamba Surabharati Prakashana Varanasi; reprint 1994; Sutra Sthana 24/9; pp 98
4. Sushruta; Sushruta Samhita; with Nibandha Sangraha commentary of Sri Dalhanacharya, edited by Yadavji Trikumji Acharya; Chaukhamba Surabharati Prakashana Varanasi; reprint 1994; Sutra sthana 24/9; pp 98
5. Agnivesha; Caraka samhita; with Ayurveda Dipika commentary by Chakrapanidatta edited by Vaidya Yadavaji Trikamji Acharya; chaukhamba Surabharati Prakashana Varanasi; reprint 2000; Chikitsa Sthana 14/6; pp 501
6. Agnivesha; Caraka samhita; with Ayurveda Dipika commentary by Chakrapanidatta edited by Vaidya Yadavaji Trikamji Acharya; chaukhamba Surabharati Prakashana Varanasi; reprint 2000; Chikitsa Sthana 14/5; pp 501
7. Devi Chand.M.A; The Atharva veda; Sanskirt text with English translation; Munshiram Manoharlal Publishers; 1997; Khanda VIII; Hymn-VI; 2153; pp 353

8. Devi Chand.M.A; The Atharva veda; Sanskirt text with English translation; Munshiram Manoharlal Publishers; 1997; Khanda VIII; Hymn-VI; 2155; pp 353

9. Agnivesha; Caraka samhita; with Ayurveda Dipika commentary by Chakrapanidatta edited by Vaidya Yadavaji Trikamji Acharya; chaukhamba Surabharati Prakashana Varanasi; reprint 2000; Chikitsa Sthana 14/12; pp 502

10. Agnivesha; Caraka samhita; with Ayurveda Dipika commentary by Chakrapanidatta edited by Vaidya Yadavaji Trikamji Acharya; chaukhamba Surabharati Prakashana Varanasi; reprint 2000; Chikitsa Sthana 14/15; pp 502

11. Agnivesha; Caraka samhita; with Ayurveda Dipika commentary by Chakrapanidatta edited by Vaidya Yadavaji Trikamji Acharya; chaukhamba Surabharati Prakashana Varanasi; reprint 2000; Chikitsa Sthana 14/19; pp 503

12. Agnivesha; Caraka samhita; with Ayurveda Dipika commentary by Chakrapanidatta edited by Vaidya Yadavaji Trikamji Acharya; chaukhamba Surabharati Prakashana Varanasi; reprint 2000; Chikitsa Sthana 14/244; pp 511

13. Vagbhata; Ashtangahridaya; with commentaries of Sarvangasundara of Arunadatta & Ayurveda rasayana of Hemadri; annoted by Dr. Anna Moreshwar Kunte & Krishna Ramachandra Shastri Narve; edited by Pt. Hari Sadashiva Shastri Paradhakar; Chaukhamba Surabharati Prakashana; reprint 2002; Nidana Sthana 7/12-13; pp 491

14. Agnivesha; Caraka samhita; with Ayurveda Dipika commentary by Chakrapanidatta edited by Vaidya Yadavaji Trikamji Acharya; chaukhamba Surabharati Prakashana Varanasi; reprint 2000; Chikitsa Sthana 14/5; pp 501

15. Sushruta; Sushruta Samhita; with Nibandha Sangraha commentary of Sri Dalhanacharya, edited by Yadavji Trikumji Acharya; Chaukhamba Surabharati Prakashana Varanasi; reprint 1994; Nidana sthana 2/4; pp 224

16. Bhavamishra; Bhavaprakasha; Vidyotini with hindi commentory by Bhishagratna Pandit Sri Brahma Sahankara Mishra; Part II; Chaukhambha Sanskrit Sansthan; 7th edition 2000; Chikitsa Prakarana 5/8; pp 46

17. Sushruta; Sushruta Samhita; with Nibandha Sangraha commentary of Sri Dalhanacharya, edited by Yadavji Trikumji Acharya; Chaukhamba Surabharati Prakashana Varanasi; reprint 1994; Nidana sthana 2/8; pp 224

18. Sushruta; Sushruta Samhita; with Nibandha Sangraha commentary of Sri Dalhanacharya, edited by Yadavji Trikumji Acharya; Chaukhamba Surabharati Prakashana Varanasi; reprint 1994; Nidana sthana 2/5-7; pp 224

19. Sushruta; Sushruta Samhita; with Nibandha Sangraha commentary of Sri Dalhanacharya, edited by Yadavji Trikumji Acharya; Chaukhamba Surabharati Prakashana Varanasi; reprint 1994; Shareera sthana 5/37; pp 285

20. Sushruta; Sushruta Samhita; with Nibandha Sangraha commentary of Sri Dalhanacharya, edited by Yadavji Trikumji Acharya; Chaukhamba Surabharati Prakashana Varanasi; reprint 1994; Nidana sthana 2/10; pp 224

21. Sushruta; Sushruta Samhita; with Nibandha Sangraha commentary of Sri Dalhanacharya, edited by Yadavji Trikumji Acharya; Chaukhamba Surabharati Prakashana Varanasi; reprint 1994; Nidana sthana 2/11; pp 224

22. Sushruta; Sushruta Samhita; with Nibandha Sangraha commentary of Sri Dalhanacharya, edited by Yadavji Trikumji Acharya; Chaukhamba Surabharati Prakashana Varanasi; reprint 1994; Nidana sthana 2/12; pp 225

23. Sushruta; Sushruta Samhita; with Nibandha Sangraha commentary of Sri Dalhanacharya, edited by Yadavji Trikumji Acharya; Chaukhamba Surabharati Prakashana Varanasi; reprint 1994; Nidana sthana 2/13; pp 225

24. Agnivesha; Caraka samhita; with Ayurveda Dipika commentary by Chakrapanidatta edited by Vaidya Yadavaji Trikamji Acharya; chaukhamba Surabharati Prakashana Varanasi; reprint 2000; Chikitsa Sthana 14/60-61; pp 504

25. Agnivesha; Caraka samhita; with Ayurveda Dipika commentary by Chakrapanidatta edited by Vaidya Yadavaji Trikamji Acharya; chaukhamba Surabharati Prakashana Varanasi; reprint 2000; Chikitsa Sthana 14/26-31; pp 503

26. Sushruta; Sushruta Samhita; with Nibandha Sangraha commentary of Sri Dalhanacharya, edited by Yadavji Trikumji Acharya; Chaukhamba Surabharati Prakashana Varanasi; reprint 1994; Chikitsa sthana 6/3; pp 343

27. Sri Vaidya Sodhala; Gada Nigraha with Vidyotini hindi commentary; by Sri Indradeva Tripathi edited by Sri Ganga Sahaya Pandeya; Part II ; Kayachikitsa Khanda;The Chowkhamba Sanskrit series office; First edition 1969; 4/53; pp 216

28. Sushruta; Sushruta Samhita; with Nibandha Sangraha commentary of Sri Dalhanacharya, edited by Yadavji Trikumji Acharya; Chaukhamba Surabharati Prakashana Varanasi; reprint 1994; Chikitsa sthana 6/16; pp 346

29. Agnivesha; Caraka samhita; with Ayurveda Dipika commentary by Chakrapanidatta edited by Vaidya Yadavaji Trikamji Acharya; chaukhamba Surabharati Prakashana Varanasi; reprint 2000; Siddi Sthana 2/13; pp 688

30. Sushruta; Sushruta Samhita; with Nibandha Sangraha commentary of Sri Dalhanacharya, edited by Yadavji Trikumji Acharya; Chaukhamba Surabharati Prakashana Varanasi; reprint 1994; Chikitsa sthana 6/13; pp 345

31. Agnivesha; Caraka samhita; with Ayurveda Dipika commentary by Chakrapanidatta edited by Vaidya Yadavaji Trikamji Acharya; chaukhamba Surabharati Prakashana Varanasi; reprint 2000; Chikitsa Sthana 14/137; pp 507

32. Agnivesha; Caraka samhita; with Ayurveda Dipika commentary by Chakrapanidatta edited by Vaidya Yadavaji Trikamji Acharya; chaukhamba Surabharati Prakashana Varanasi; reprint 2000; Siddi Sthana 3/38-42; pp 696

33. Bhela – Samhita; text with English translation; commentary and critical notes by Dr. K.H.Krishnamurthy, edited by Prof. Priya Vrat Sharma; Chaukhambha Visvabharathi, Varanasi; 1st edition; Chikitsa sthana; 16/86; pp 407

34. Vagbhata; Ashtangahridaya; with commentaries of Sarvangasundara of Arunadatta & Ayurveda rasayana of Hemadri; annoted by Dr. Anna Moreshwar Kunte & Krishna Ramachandra Shastri Narve; edited by Pt. Hari Sadashiva Shastri Paradhakar; Chaukhamba Surabharati Prakashana; reprint 2002; Chikitsa Sthana 8/88; pp 649

35. Vagbhata; Ashtangasangraha; with Hindi commentary by Kaviraj Atrideva Gupta; Krishnadasa Academy; reprint 1993; Chikitsa Sthana 10/9; pp 61

36. Agnivesha; Caraka samhita; with Ayurveda Dipika commentary by Chakrapanidatta edited by Vaidya Yadavaji Trikamji Acharya; chaukhamba Surabharati Prakashana Varanasi; reprint 2000; Chikitsa Sthana 14/175; 176; 183; pp 508 - 509

37. Vagbhata; Ashtangasangraha; with Hindi commentary by Kaviraj Atrideva Gupta; Krishnadasa Academy; reprint 1993; Chikitsa Sthana 10/32; pp 64

38. Sushruta; Sushruta Samhita; with Nibandha Sangraha commentary of Sri Dalhanacharya, edited by Yadavji Trikumji Acharya; Chaukhamba Surabharati Prakashana Varanasi; reprint 1994; Chikitsa sthana 6/11; pp 344

39. Vagbhata; Ashtangasangraha; with Hindi commentary by Kaviraj Atrideva Gupta; Krishnadasa Academy; reprint 1993; Chikitsa Sthana 10/58; pp 68

40. Sushruta; Sushruta Samhita; with Nibandha Sangraha commentary of Sri Dalhanacharya, edited by Yadavji Trikumji Acharya; Chaukhamba Surabharati Prakashana Varanasi; reprint 1994; Chikitsa sthana 6/3; pp 343

41. Sushruta; Sushruta Samhita; with Nibandha Sangraha commentary of Sri Dalhanacharya, edited by Yadavji Trikumji Acharya; Chaukhamba Surabharati Prakashana Varanasi; reprint 1994; Chikitsa sthana 6/4; pp 343

42. Vagbhata; Ashtangasangraha; with Hindi commentary by Kaviraj Atrideva Gupta; Krishnadasa Academy; reprint 1993; Chikitsa Sthana 10/3; pp 60

43. Sushruta; Sushruta Samhita; with Nibandha Sangraha commentary of Sri Dalhanacharya, edited by Yadavji Trikumji Acharya; Chaukhamba Surabharati Prakashana Varanasi; reprint 1994; Chikitsa sthana 6/3; pp 343

44. Vagbhata; Ashtangasangraha; Saroja Hindi Commentary by Dr. Ravidutt Tripathi; Chaukhambha Sanskrit Prathishtana Varanasi; Sutra Sthana 40/5; pp 667

45. Sushruta; Sushruta Samhita; with Nibandha Sangraha commentary of Sri Dalhanacharya, edited by Yadavji Trikumji Acharya; Chaukhamba Surabharati Prakashana Varanasi; reprint 1994; Sutra sthana 12/8; pp 45

46. Sushruta; Sushruta Samhita; with Nibandha Sangraha commentary of Sri Dalhanacharya, edited by Yadavji Trikumji Acharya; Chaukhamba Surabharati Prakashana Varanasi; reprint 1994; Chikitsa sthana 6/3; pp 343

47. Sushruta; Sushruta Samhita; with Nibandha Sangraha commentary of Sri Dalhanacharya, edited by Yadavji Trikumji Acharya; Chaukhamba Surabharati Prakashana Varanasi; reprint 1994; Chikitsa sthana 6/7; pp 344

48. Sushruta; Sushruta Samhita; with Nibandha Sangraha commentary of Sri Dalhanacharya, edited by Yadavji Trikumji

Acharya; Chaukhamba Surabharati Prakashana Varanasi; reprint 1994; Chikitsa sthana 6/10; pp 344

49. B.D.Chaurasia; Human Anatomy; CBS Publications & distributors;2nd edition 1991; pp 335-338

ABOUT THE AUTHORS

Professor (Dr.) Vivekanand Mohan Kullolli, M.S(Ayurved) & LLB, is a consulting Ayurvedic Surgeon and an academician since last 20 years. His clinical practices are more focused on the **Medical Management of Surgical Diseases**. In the Last 20 years, he has served in the different positions of academic line as Medical Superintendent to Principal, of different Ayurvedic Institutions. He is also an expert in the non-materialistic healing like **Neuro-Linguistic Programming** and **Numerology**. Presently he is working as a Professor and Researcher in the **Parul University, Vadodara, Gujarat, India** and also pursuing his doctoral (PhD) studies in the Ayurved. He is the student of **Astrology** and ***Vastu Shastra.*** He has Published more than 20 Research Papers and guided 11 Post Graduate Thesis, in the field of Ayurveda. His Aim is to create, a Series of Ayurveda Books to help, the Non Ayurvedic people also, to understand the Natural Life Science and Use it in their day-to-day life, to achieve healthy long life and Success in their respective fields.

For any queries he can be contacted through his mobile number +919945079276 and email: vivekanandkullolli@gmail.com

Dr. Krishna Thorat Kullolli, M.D (Ayu) & (PhD), is An Ayurvedic Academician, serving as an Associate Professor in the Department of ***Roga Nidan evam Vikruti Vijnanam*** (Department concerned with the study of Aetiology & Pathology in Ayurveda), **Parul Institute of Ayurved and Research, Parul University, Vadodara, Gujarat, India.** She is keen on developing the best & easy Ayurvedic diagnostic formats based on the Modern Diagnostic Tools, for the understanding of more complex chronic diseases. Her area of interest is to evaluate and incorporate the modern diagnostic tools and investigations to understand the Ayurvedic Evaluation of the Disease pathology and bridge the gap between the *Roga Nidana* (Ayurvedic way of understanding the disease pathology) and Modern Pathological Science. She is Awarded with Best Scientific Paper presentation in many National and International Seminars and Webinars, because of her unique and most appropriate approach towards Ayurvedic Pathological Principles.

Her email Id for any communication in regard to Ayurvedic Pathologies is krishthorat88@gmail.com.

Disclaimer

Health advice, medical information and treatment options which may be provided in this book are not here meant to replace any sort of professional advice.

It is best to consult with your medical practitioner or health care provider before trying out any strategies listed here.

www.ingramcontent.com/pod-product-compliance
Lightning Source LLC
LaVergne TN
LVHW010601160826
845677LV00013B/3205

* 9 7 8 9 3 9 3 3 8 8 9 5 7 *